WHAT'S NEW

IN

ALLERGY

AND

ASTHMA

Other Books by the Author

Hidden Food Allergies; How to Find and
Overcome Them Successfully

Take Charge of Your Health: Professional Secrets
You Need to Know to Obtain the Best Medical
Care

Empty Your Bucket: A Step-By-Step Method To
Control Allergy And Allergic Asthma

FOURTH EDITION, UPDATED AND REVISED

WHAT'S NEW

IN

ALLERGY

AND

ASTHMA

NEW DEVELOPMENTS
AND HOW THEY
HELP YOU OVERCOME
ALLERGY AND ASTHMA

STEPHEN ASTOR, M.D.

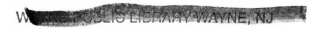

Copyright © 1996 by Stephen H. Astor

All rights reserved. No part of this publication may be reproduced, stored in a retrieval system or transmitted, in any form or by any means, electronic, mechanical, photocopying, recording, or otherwise, without the prior written permission of the copyright owner. Address inquiries to Two A's Industries, Inc., Suite 1, 285 South Drive, Mountain View, CA, 94040-4318

Printed in the United States of America.

10 9 8 7 6 5 4 3 2 1

Cataloging Data

Astor, Stephen, date.
  What's New In Allergy and Asthma.
        288p.   22.6cm.
  Index.
  1. Health   2. Self-care, Health   3. Medicine, Popular
  4. Consumer education   5. Medical care   6. Alternative medicine.
  number   1996   616.97   96-90200
ISBN 0915001128

Table of Contents

x

Introduction

Mitch was an eager college student who graduated from a university, entered a training program for stockbrokers, and thought he was doing well until he went to his first review with the woman who ran the training program. She told Mitch she was pleased with his progress but she had unexpected words of advice.

"Mitch," she said, "you're learning quickly, but you have a problem. You're constantly blowing your nose and clearing your throat. This makes a bad impression on clients who look to you for financial guidance."

"I can't help myself," Mitch replied. "I have bad allergies. I'm allergic to everything."

"Well," the director said, "you need to get treatment."

"What's the use?" Mitch answered. "Allergy treatment hasn't changed in years. They can't cure you."

Like Mitch, many people believe there is nothing new in allergy. The facts are quite the opposite. There has been an explosion of information about advanced allergy medication, how to give more effective allergy injections, new understanding about food allergy, and simplified techniques to avoid allergenic substances. This book, which is the fourth edition of *What's New in Allergy and Asthma*, describes the pros and cons of the latest developments and shows you how to use the new findings to help you control allergy.

You may wonder why it's important for you to learn the ins and outs of allergy when your doctor is supposed to read about the latest research and tell you what to do. Unfortunately, allergy treatment doesn't work this way. Each person has a unique metabolism and a unique set of allergies. Therefore each person's treatment needs to be tailored to his individual circumstances. Doctors can advise you, but you need to observe your body's response and with your doctor's help determine whether the treatment is satisfactory.

Thus, allergy treatment is a cooperative effort between you and your doctor. The more you know, the better you can follow your doctor's advice, know what to look for, and know what to report.

Another reason you need to learn about allergy is so that you can sort out the information you will come across on radio and TV, in newspapers and magazines, from friends and relatives, and from drug company advertisements. Radio, TV, newspapers, and magazines want to grab your attention. Drug companies want you to buy their products. Your friends and relatives want to be as helpful as they can. Even your doctor means well. But no one, not radio, TV, newspapers, magazines, drug companies, friends, relatives, or even your doctor can know exactly how you will respond. So, in a sense, you are on your own.

> *The allergy treatment that helps one person cannot be guaranteed to help another person.*

> *Your best bet to control your allergy is to learn as much as you can about allergy, consider the various options, and work with your doctor to figure out what treatment is best for you.*

This book explains the significant developments in the field of allergy in easy to understand language. You may read the entire book or simply turn to the section that fits your case.

The book is divided into chapters. Each chapter contains several reports. Each report describes the results of experiments that have been performed by experts in the field of allergy. To give you an example of how many thousands of research projects have been completed, I can tell you that for the past five years scientists of the American Academy of Allergy, Asthma, and Immunology have completed over nine hundred experiments *each year*. And the American Academy of Allergy, Asthma, and Immunology is just one of many allergy associations. There are also the American College of Allergy, the Association for the Care of Asthma, and the National Institutes for Lung and Respiratory Diseases, to name just a few.

Since this book is for the layperson, you won't read about complex, biochemical reactions. Instead you will learn practical steps about how and when to use new drugs, ways to improve the effectiveness of allergy injections, measures that you can adopt that have been found helpful in preventing allergies, and certain diseases whose origins were unknown but, upon investigation, turned out to be caused by allergy. Equally important for you, and often overlooked, are studies which show the limitations and *disadvantages* of certain allergy treatments that were once thought to be useful and have been shown to be ineffective or dangerous.

You will learn that allergy is not a deficiency or weakness but an overabundance of an antibody called IgE antibody. The chapters on environmental allergens such as dust, dust mite, pets and mold will teach you simple techniques to avoid allergens so you can prevent allergy symptoms before they start. New to this edition are chapters on alternative treatments and asthma. There are also tips on how to obtain allergy treatment if you belong to a managed care insurance plan.

There is a lot of information packed into these pages. Some of it is so new your doctors may not even know about it. Physicians who are in clinical practice often don't have the time to read about advances in *every* specialty of medicine. That is why we have specialists who concentrate on a particular field. If your doctor wants to know more about a particular topic, I included the name of at least one of the scientists who did the original research. Your doctor will be able to read the original experiment if he or she wishes.

At the end of each report there are helpful hints to aid you in putting the information into perspective. An allergy treatment that applies to a woman may not apply to a man. A treatment that works in a child may not help an adult. An injection that works for pollens may not help for foods. A technique that seems to cure allergy quickly may have long-term side effects.

Unfortunately, there isn't a universal answer that fits every situation.

Know What You Are Doing To Your Body

When you suffer from a chronic disease such as allergy, you must learn the advantages and disadvantages of your treatments. You may not like what you hear, however. Sometimes the truth is hard to take. But it is better to face the facts from the beginning. Where your health is concerned, improper treatment can be more than a mere disappointment. It can actually harm you!

What's New in Allergy and Asthma is an adventure. Your trip will unmask myths, teach you surprising facts, and help *you*, the allergy sufferer, get the most from modern medicine.

1

What Is Allergy? How Do People Get Allergy? How Do I Learn About My Own Allergy?

There are a lot of myths and misunderstandings about how people develop allergy. Over the years I've heard them all. You may have heard them, too. Some say allergy is a weakness or deficiency of the immune system. Others say allergy is due to a lack of vitamins, too much histamine, or chronic infections.

Although there are many different ideas about what causes allergy, most people react the same way upon being told they *have* allergy. "I don't believe it," they reply. "How could I suddenly be allergic to a substance I've been exposed to or a food I've eaten my whole life?"

These and questions about when to seek help, what kind of doctor to see, and what constitutes an allergy work-up are answered in this chapter. The first report comes from data that was collected by the National Institutes of Health. Look at the table and you can see where you stand in relation to others who have allergy. When you add the numbers it's quite amazing how many people suffer.

The next studies explain how allergies begin and how they run in families. After doctors understood this, they turned their attention to devising a way to prevent allergies. The next study describes the results of an experiment that was done in the expectation that you might be able to prevent allergy by breast-feeding children. Next is a study that tells you what doctors and insurance companies learned when they tried to assess how allergy compromised quality of life.

The next group of studies tell you how an allergy work up can be completed in one visit and, in a section titled 'Will the Real Allergist Please Stand Up!', what kind of doctor to consult. Then there are studies explaining how important it is to see a specialist, what treatments allergy offers, the worst allergy location in the United States, and the worst year for allergy sufferers.

With this background information you are on your way to understanding the newer developments and learning how to use them to control your allergies. This will lead to a healthier you.

How Many People Suffer Like I Do?

According to the National Institutes of Health, which is the Department of the United States government that is responsible for overseeing the scientific aspects of health care in America, millions of people suffer with allergy. The following figures are from recent years and are based on a total population of approximately 250 million people. You can see where you fit in by looking at the type of allergy you have in the left-hand column and seeing how many people have the same condition.

Prevelance of Allergic Diseases in the United States-1993

Hayfever and Allergic rhinitis:	24.2 million people
Asthma	15 million people 5,000 deaths per year 500,000 hospital admissions $6.2 billion dollars cost of treatment
Sinusitis	32.2 million people
Food allergy	8% children below 6 years 2% of adults
Insect sting allergy	1-5% of population 40 deaths per year
Hives	15% of population
Eczema	4-10% of children
Medication reactions	70,000 reported to the Food and Drug Administration. (Millions more are too insignificant to report.)

Helpful hint 1: I'm sure you don't need me to tell you this, but if you have allergy, you aren't alone.

Helpful hint 2: Just because there are millions of people who suffer like you and even if many of them are worse off than you, this does not mean you need to suffer, too. Take the time and trouble to learn how to feel better. You won't win an award for being a martyr.

Now We Understand Why People Suddenly Develop Allergies

You may be puzzled about how you could suddenly be allergic to a dog you've had for ten years or a cheese you've been eating for twenty years. The symptoms seem to appear out of the clear blue sky. And because there were no prior indications of allergy, you may not believe this could be happening to you.

Although the seemingly sudden onset of symptoms may seem unique to allergy, sudden onset occurs with many diseases. Cancer, heart conditions, and ulcer are typical examples. These illnesses develop over a period of time. However you only become aware of them at a *specific point* in time.

It is the same story with allergic disorders. Certain people are *predisposed* to allergy due to a flaw in their ability to regulate the level of an antibody called IgE. Because of this flaw, they *eventually* make *too much* IgE. Slowly and surely and after repeated exposure to various substances, their level of IgE rises. When their IgE has reached a level that is excessive, the actual symptoms begin. Dr. Rebecca Buckley of Duke University studied IgE and confirmed that allergy is due to excess IgE antibody.

> *Once IgE hits an excess level, the symptoms of allergy begin.*

Those of you who manufacture IgE very fast will reach an excess level early in your life and therefore you will develop allergies when you are young. Those of you who manufacture IgE more slowly might take fifteen or twenty years to reach an excess level. Some of you, and this is true of the majority of individuals, manufacture IgE at the normal rate and, lucky you, you *never* develop allergies.

Exposure Needed For Allergy To Develop

There is an additional fact you need to know to help you understand why allergies take time to develop. Your body won't make antibodies unless it is exposed to a particular substance. For example, if you *never* take penicillin, you cannot become allergic to penicillin. However, if your body has the tendency or predisposition to make too much IgE antibody *and* if you take a lot of penicillin, chances are you will eventually wind up allergic to penicillin. The same is true for exposure to grasses, weeds, trees, dust, and dogs.

In fact, when it comes to determining what is most likely responsible for the apparent sudden onset of allergic symptoms, most allergists are more suspicious of substances you have been exposed to throughout your life than something that is brand new in your life.

Helpful hint 1: Allergies develop over a period of time after repeated exposure in certain susceptible individuals.

Helpful hint 2: Two thirds of people manufacture IgE antibody at the *normal* rate. No matter how often these individuals are exposed to allergenic substances they *never* become allergic. Population studies show that the *remaining* one-third of the population has allergy. In these studies, though, allergy is defined in strict medical terms (i.e. excess IgE). People who are allergic to work or their spouse don't count!

Helpful hint 3: Even though one third of people develop allergy, many cases are mild and do not need extensive treatment. So you do not need to be paranoid about developing allergy.

How Allergies Run In Families

As you may have heard, allergies tend to occur in families. This is because the difficulty in regulating IgE antibody is usually an *inherited* characteristic.

Interestingly, though, members of a family don't inherit allergy to *identical* substances. Instead, what they become allergic to depends on their lifestyle and habits because lifestyle and habits determine what allergens you are exposed to.

Dr. Sami Bahna thought it would be a good idea to study twins to learn more about how *specific* allergies run in families.

Studies Of Twins

Dr. Bahna showed that if one twin had allergies, the other did too. However, the *specific* allergens that each twin had become allergic to and the way those allergens were affecting them was different.

If one twin was allergic to grasses and weeds, the other could be allergic to dogs and cats. One to foods and the other to dust. To make it more confusing, if both twins were allergic to dog dander, in one the dog could provoke sneezing and in the other it could provoke wheezing. Peanuts could cause hives in one twin, while in the other peanuts might provoke gastrointestinal symptoms. There was no way Dr. Bahna could predict how one twin would react no matter how extensively he studied the other.

Dr. Bahna's research is a good reminder that when individuals inherit allergy, they inherit the *ability to become allergic* and not allergy to a specific substance.

Helpful hint 1: The *predisposition* to develop allergy runs in families. Allergy to a *specific substance* is determined by *your* exposure to that substance.

Helpful hint 2: You cannot skin test one member of a family in order to learn about the allergies of other members of the family.

Can Breast Feeding Prevent Allergies?

Since doctors know that allergy is caused by *exposure to a specific substance* and the *inherited tendency to make excessive IgE*, they theorized that by removing the exposure side of the equation they might be able to prevent the accumulation of excess IgE.

To investigate this, Dr. Robert Hamburger from San Diego studied breast-feeding. Dr. Hamburger divided his mothers into two groups. Some breast-fed their babies, and some did not. If the breast-fed children had grown up free of allergy, the answer would have been clear-cut. Breast-feeding would have been proven to prevent allergy. However, when the results were in, some of the children who were breast-fed got allergy anyway. Further confusing the issue was the fact that some of the bottle-fed children who would have been expected to get allergy did *not* get allergy.

When you think about how complicated the allergic process is, you would expect this sort of result. Since it takes exposure *and* susceptibility to produce allergy, removing only *one* of the factors, the exposure to cows' milk, would simply *delay* an infant's exposure and subsequent sensitization. Breast-feeding could not be expected to *prevent* allergy to milk *forever*. Even if avoiding cows' milk was successful in preventing allergy to cows' milk, this would not prevent a child's exposure to other foods. Nor would it prevent exposure to dust, grasses, or a family dog. The child, therefore, could still become allergic to these allergens.

Aside from the theoretical arguments against breast feeding as a way to prevent allergy, the most telling blow and the most important consideration was that the experiment did not work.

The basic defect in allergy is an *inherited* characteristic, much like the color of your eyes is an inherited characteristic. I need not remind you that you cannot change your inheritance by changing your diet.

Additionally, in a more recent study of nursing mothers who drank cows' milk when they were breast feeding, Dr. S. Giordano showed that allergenic components of cows' milk passed into the breast milk. Thus these mothers' infants were being exposed to cows' milk even though it seemed that they were only eating breast milk. If such an infant is predisposed to make too much IgE, the infant can become sensitized.

Helpful hint 1: Breast-feeding will not prevent an infant's exposure to cows' milk if the mother eats cows' milk or cows' milk products. Cows' milk protein will pass into the child through the breast milk and can sensitize the child.

Helpful hint 2: Breast-feeding does not prevent or delay exposure to other allergens such as dogs, cats, dust, pollens, and other foods. Even if it could, you cannot keep your babies in protective custody for their whole life.

Helpful hint 3: Whether you breast-feed or not, only one third of children develop allergy anyway.

Helpful hint 4: If your child develops allergy, you can begin treatment at any time. Usually, treatment requires only a few simple changes in the environment.

Helpful hint 5: If you want to breast feed your infant because you enjoy it, go right ahead. If you are breast-feeding to prevent allergies, you should reconsider your decision.

Quality of Life with Allergy

Many people, including certain doctors, consider allergy a nuisance and not a disease. This is a shortsighted view and not consonant with the facts. Allergy can maim you from secondary infections, excess fatigue, lost work, missed shool, and inability to function at your best. It can put you in the hospital with asthma or anaphylaxis. And it can kill you through uncontrolled asthma, a fatal food, drug, or insect-sting reaction, or even an automobile fatality from falling asleep at the wheel due to using an allergy drug that causes drowsiness. So while allergy *usually* isn't a severe disease like cancer and is *often* a mere nuisance like a few sneezes once in a while, allergy isn't a piece of cake, either.

How do you measure quality of life so you can tell whether you should seek treatment or grin and bear it? Over the past few years doctors and certain patients have been working with managed care insurance companies to establish guidelines that measure quality of life so they can assess various treatments. You can use the same guidelines to figure out what impact allergy is having on *your* quality of life.

The first task was to define the problem, and the following statements were used to do this. The statements were made to researchers who were conducting studies at various teaching institutions. The investigators utilized members of an allergy support group called The National Allergy and Asthma Network/Mothers of Asthmatics. While these patients' allergies weren't necessarily life-threatening, they interfered with their own or their children's lives. If one of the statements sounds familiar, discuss this with your health care provider.

The principal investigator of one of the studies is Richard Schulz, Ph.D., who is a professor at the College of Pharmacy at the University of South Carolina. Below are the kinds of things that Dr. Schulz found.

Adults

• I am torn between my need for freedom and my need to do, eat, and go where I want.

• I have had to change my work or my work schedule because of allergy.

• I keep falling behind in work because I'm too ill to function.

• Allergy medication makes me work slower.

•I feel there is something wrong with me because I'm so vulnerable.

•I am physically and emotionally worn down trying to treat allergy attacks.

•I am jealous of people who don't have to worry about allergy.

•I'm upset with doctors because they can't cure me.

•Housework is a non-stop chore due to allergy.

•I have to watch everything I eat because of allergy.

•I can't go in the garden because of allergy.

•I'm afraid to swim because there are stinging bees around the pool.

•Allergy adds tension to my marriage.

•The cost of care is a burden, and it's unfair that I have to suffer with allergy and have to pay so much to feel better.

•I worry that allergy medicine will have long-term effects, and I resent having to take so much.

•These drugs work, but the side effects are killing me.

•Every time I get a cold I'm on medicine for weeks. Why can't I get a cold that last two-days like everyone else?

•I (or my child) would accomplish more if not for allergy and asthma.

•I am uncomfortable going to a friend's or relative's house where I (or my child) may be exposed to allergens that make me sick.

•I feel like I need to live in a glass bubble.

•I feel that people think I'm strange because of all the precautions I need to take.

•I keep getting secondary sinus, bronchitis, and ear infections because of my underlying allergy.

•I spend half my life at the doctor's office.

Children

•I struggle to balance my child's need for freedom and my need to protect against allergic reactions.

•I tend to be overprotective of my child.

•I have responsibilities to my allergic child and feel badly when I can't spend time with my other children.

•The teachers at school do their best, but they don't have the experience to take care of my child like I can during an acute attack.

Helpful hint 1: Quality of life can be difficult to measure because each person has different standards. You have to define *your own standards* and not leave this up to an insurance company, your friends, or your boss.

Helpful hint 2: If you have to deal with a managed care insurance company which is reluctant to authorize allergy treatment for you, write to the medical director and explain what quality of life means to you and how your symptoms prevent you from achieving the quality of life you desire. Otherwise, the company might be tempted to use a dollars-and-cents analysis in their favor when deciding how much care they wish to provide for you.

Helpful hint 3: Although we medical doctors like to think we are the only ones who can do useful medical research, sometimes we can learn from astute researchers in other fields such as the work done by Dr. Schulz who is a professor in a school of pharmacy.

The One-Visit Allergy Workup

Did you ever wonder why allergists ask you to come for multiple appointments for a complete allergy workup? Typically the doctor obtains a history at the first appointment. At subsequent appointments he performs skin tests. Finally he explains the results and tells you what to do. At some offices, you don't even get to see the allergist until the final visit. A nurse does the work.

When I was in training, my professors scheduled an hour appointment and we had to complete the workup in one visit. This made sense in training because it saved time and money. It still makes sense.

Although it is traditional to have several visits for a complete allergy evaluation, there isn't a scientific reason to do this. A doctor can take a complete history, do tests by the grouping method (see How to Cut the Cost of An Allergy Workup), and tell you the results in one visit.

Helpful hint 1: There isn't a medical law that says you must make several visits over a period of many weeks to have a complete allergy workup.

Will The Real Allergist Please Stand Up?

When you decide to consult a doctor for allergy treatment, you have to choose between doctors who are Board Certified in Allergy and Immunology and those who aren't. The distinction is based on the amount and thoroughness of training your health care professional obtained.

Since many allergy problems aren't complex, you may not require a health care professional who has complete training. In the United States there are only about 4,000 Board Certified allergists anyway. They couldn't possibly see everyone who has allergy. Statistics show that one-third of the population (over seventy million people) have allergy. Thus, chances are that you will have to obtain your allergy care from someone who isn't Board Certified.

Like many people you may be embarrassed to ask whether your doctor is Board Certified, what kind of training he has had, and whether he is qualified to handle your case. People who would not hesitate to ask their auto mechanic these basic questions are too timid to ask when it comes to their own body.

On the other hand, you may not need a fully-trained professional. Some allergy problems are obvious. If you have hives after you eat peanuts, you do not need a Board Certified Allergist to help you. A good friend might figure this out and tell you to stop eating peanuts. However, while the advice is correct this does not qualify your friend as an allergist.

Beware of Phonies

You must beware of phonies. Many health care providers practice allergy and some even call themselves allergists even though they haven't been trained. Insurance companies created another problem when they entered the managed care business. They often decide you must make several visits to a Primary Care Doctor before they allow you to see a specialist. This can be penny-wise and pound-foolish. A doctor who has spent his life studying a particular disease can usually diagnose and prescribe a solution faster and in many cases cheaper than a non-specialist. Nevertheless managed care is here to stay.

Certified Allergists

To become Board Certified in allergy, a physician must study three to four years to become Board Certified in Internal Medicine, Pediatrics, or Family Practice. Then the physician must study two *additional* years in one of fifty special allergy programs in the United States or Canada. Upon satisfactory completion of the allergy training program, the doctor must pass a written and oral examination in allergy. Upon successful completion of the exams, the physician is given the designation Board Certified in Allergy and Immunology.

To learn whether a physician is Board Certified, you may write to the American Board of Allergy and Immunology, University Science Center, 3624 Market St., Philadelphia, PA, 19104.

Uncertified Allergists

Unlike Board Certified Allergists, where there is one kind of certification, there are *three* types of uncertified allergist.

First, there are health care providers such as Family Practitioners, Pediatricians, Ear, Nose and Throat Surgeons, Internists, Chiropractors and Acupuncturists. These professionals must learn a little about everything, including allergy, in order to take care of their patients.

It will not be easy for you to decide whether a problem can be handled by your Family Practitioner, Pediatrician, or Chiropractor, or whether you ought to see a Board Certified Allergist. This is a decision *you* must make. You are the person who has the problem. You must decide what is in your best interest. If you are part of a managed care insurance plan, you may even have to appeal, in writing, to the plan's medical director.

If you are one of the many people who are afraid to hurt your Primary Care Doctor's feelings by asking him for a referral to a specialist or who assume your doctor would initiate a referral if he felt you needed one, you must overcome this feeling. Some doctors wait for their patients to request a referral on the assumption that if the symptoms were bothersome the patient would ask to see a specialist. This you-go-first scenario reminds me of two people who enter an elevator together. Each one waits for the other. Meanwhile the doors close and it is too late for either one to get on.

The second group of health care professionals who are not Board Certified in allergy, but nevertheless practice allergy, are clinical ecologists and doctors who specialize in environmental medicine. These people are trained by other ecologists because medical schools do not offer this type of instruction. The tests these professionals use such as cytotoxic, sublingual, and certain muscle tests and the treatments they prescribe such as injections of chemicals, neutralizing shots and sublingual drops have proved to be unreliable in the vast majority of cases.

You may see newspaper articles about environmental medicine and clinical ecology and how modern chemicals are poisonous. You may hear dramatic, personal testimonials about how ecological-environmental treament has helped sufferers. However, *controlled* studies show that few people benefit. Yet the few successful cases give everyone hope and make them ignore the statistics.

One area where ecology treatment can help is in the area of *toxic, irritant* chemicals that are in the air from *excessive* levels of fumes, vapors, gases, and particles that are part of our industrialized society. The treatment is avoidance because immunizing injections don't work for toxic exposures.

Finally the third group of uncertified allergists consists of your friends, neighbors, relatives, and pharmacists. Allergy is a common problem. Everyone seems to have an opinion about it. Sometimes their opinion is correct. Sometimes it isn't. You can judge by the results. If a friend's opinion to stop eating peanuts solves your problem, you may not need further advice. If your problem isn't solved, you should seek *expert* help.

Interestingly, the cost of an allergy workup and subsequent treatment is frequently inversely related to the quality and thoroughness of your doctor's training. Ecologists often perform expensive testing using cytotoxic, neutralizing technique, sublingual drops, and total environmental isolation. Their charges can run from $2,000 to $10,000. In contrast, charges for a Board Certified allergist usually run $575 to $750 for a complete workup, including testing and the final summary visit.

It may seem contradictory that doctors who have less training charge more money. However, these physicians rely on highly expensive and inaccurate tests instead of the medical history, a physical examination, clinical experience, and common sense. Patients often forget that a test, no matter how modern or heavily advertised it may be, is not infallible. The test must be interpreted correctly. For example, a blood pressure of 60/40 might be normal in a small, thin child who was lying in bed. In an adult, this pressure indicates cardiovascular shock. A hemoglobin of eighteen might be normal in an individual who lives on a mountain where the air is thin. At sea level this indicates a blood disease.

In an era where so many sophisticated tests are available, you probably want to have the latest ones performed on you. However, unless you have a scientific background, you may not be in a position to judge the usefulness and accuracy of certain tests.

Even doctors are human and can be swayed by advertising. Unless your doctors have the time to read the scientific literature carefully, they can fall into the same trap as if *you* rely on newspaper stories, magazine articles, and advertising for your medical advice. Food tests are a perfect example. Skin, blood, sublingual drop, muscle, and neutralizing tests are inaccurate. But they are heavily promoted. Although these tests aren't dangerous, they don't give reliable answers. Yet, many physicians may feel pressured into ordering them. Unaware of the high frequency of false positive and false negative results, they may make the mistake of assuming a positive test always indicates a cause and effect relationship.

I have met Board Certified allergists who were swayed by the seductive advertising of companies that promote blood tests for food allergy. If they can be convinced by high pressure ads, think how easy it is to convince the non-specialist and even easier to convince a layperson.

Choosing an allergist is the same as choosing someone to service your car, your television, or your taxes. You can go to a person who is self-taught, has a moderate degree of training, or is fully trained. Whomever you choose, you may get lucky. But your chance for a successful outcome is better if you consult someone who has been *properly* trained.

Helpful hint 1: There are many health care professionals offering allergy advice. You need to think of your own interests when deciding whom to consult.

Helpful hint 2: I have never met a doctor who was mad at a patient when the patient asked to see a specialist.

Helpful hint 3: I have never met a managed care plan that automatically sent its patients to a specialist for allergy treatment. You need to ask.

Helpful hint 4: Do not confuse reactions to toxic, irritant chemicals with allergy to natural substances like foods, plants, animals, and housedust.

Talk to Me, Doctor

E. Horowitz and several associates from Baltimore found that doctors tend to discuss the causes and treatment of allergy with parents and guardians of children instead of the children themselves. This occurred even when the children were of high school age. This left the children unaware of what caused their problem and what they could do about it.

The researchers concluded that health care professionals should communicate with the patient, *no matter how young the person is*. After all, the allergy sufferer must learn when and how to adjust his activities, manage his medication, and give feedback to his doctor. He is the first one to know when he is getting worse and is thus the first to be able to intervene early when the symptoms are more likely to respond. To do this, though, he needs to be educated.

Dr. C. Szelc Kelly studied children at a summer camp for asthmatics, and Dr. A. J. Althaus studied children who were given in-home education. Both doctors discovered that good education reduced the number of emergency room visits, office visits, hospital admissions, and school absences. The net savings in dollars was an astounding $2,000 per child, in addition to enabling each child to live a happier and more productive life.

> **Helpful hint 1**: Although it is tempting to discuss allergy treatment with the parents when the patient is a child on the theory that children can't be trusted, several doctors have shown that children can learn and be trusted. They need to be included in the discussion and made part of the management team *from the beginning*. This can be accomplished through in-home education and attendance at special asthma camps, in addition to the usual education in the doctor's office.

The Three Treatments For Allergy

One of the most unusual concepts for me to explain about allergy is that you, the patient, must help in selecting your treatment. I wrote about this in *Take Charge of Your Health*. It's worth repeating here.

Allergy is different from many fields of medicine. In other fields there is often a single treatment. For example, for appendicitis, you need an operation. For a strep throat, you need an antibiotic. For diabetes, you need insulin. For allergy, though, there are *three* choices. Avoid what you are allergic to, take medicine to alleviate the symptoms, or start allergy injections to build your immunity. Your choice will depend on what you are allergic to, what you are able to do, and how your body responds to medication.

To figure out what to do, you must consider all the factors, such as your lifestyle, age, hobbies, family, and type of work. So before deciding on a course of treatment, consider how that treatment fits *your* situation. For personal, medical, or fanciful reasons, you may prefer one treatment over another.

Let's look at the three options for allergy.

Avoidance

The best treatment for allergy is avoidance. Although avoidance always works, this may not be the most practical solution for you. Depending on your lifestyle and occupation, avoidance may not even be possible.

Medication

The second method of treatment is use of medication. Generally, modern medicines work well, and we have been able to reduce many of the side effects. However, in certain individuals, even modern medicines produce side effects which are sometimes worse than the original problem. Common side effects of allergy drugs are nervousness, jitteriness, and drowsiness. Another problem with medication is that you may take so much medication that your body builds a resistance or immunity to the drug. Another problem is that certain drugs don't work in certain people. The biggest problem with allergy medicine is that they do not cure the underlying condition. They just relieve the symptoms.

Don't let the fact that modern allergy medications do not cure allergy discourage you from using them. There are not many diseases where drugs do cure. As you know, insulin, anti-hypertensive drugs, and arthritis medications merely provide temporary relief. We accept this limitation because temporary relief is better than no relief.

Immunizing Injections

The third type of allergy treatment is the use of immunizing injections. Immunization is a long process, but in the end your resistance is boosted. Just as your family doctor can increase your resistance to measles, mumps, polio, and flu by giving you injections of measles, mumps, polio and flu, an allergist can increase your resistance to grasses, trees, weeds, dust, pets, and mold by injecting you with grasses, trees, weeds, dust, pets, and mold.

You start with a low dose and build up. Using the high dose method, you get injections once or twice week for ten to twenty weeks. You continue the shots with a monthly maintenance dose for about three years. Generally speaking, at the end of three years you will have enough permanent immunity so that you can stop the shots. The schedule may vary depending on your particular allergies, but you rarely need to be on shots "forever."

Some offices use the *low dose* injection method. On the low dose regimens, you need more injections, more often, and for more years than I just described. Low dose isn't right or wrong. It just takes longer.

Finally, when it comes to allergy treatments, you have a fourth choice. This is cortisone-steroids. Cortisone-steroid is a drug, and strictly speaking it should be in the medication category. I consider cortisone separately because it can cause long-term, serious side effects such as weight gain, high blood pressure, ulcer, cataracts, softening of bones, stunting growth in children, and psychological changes. Thus, I think of cortisone-steroid separately and prefer to use this kind of medication *only* when the other measures don't work.

Sometimes it is hard to know if you are taking cortisone-steroid. For example, your doctor may prescribe Medrol. You probably would not know that Medrol is a brand of cortisone-steroid. Or you may be given an "allergy shot" in the nose. Nine times out of ten an allergy shot in the nose is an injection of cortisone-steroid. Even a nasal spray may be called by a different name, thus disguising the fact that it is cortisone-based.

The Allergist's Duty

An allergist's primary job is to help you figure out which of the three choices of treatment is most suitable *for your particular case*. The answer depends on many factors. This detective work makes allergy interesting. No two cases are alike. Even if your allergies are identical to another person's, your treatment might be different because you have a different lifestyle, occupation, hobby, and so forth. This is why you need to take charge of your health when it comes to allergy.

Helpful hint 1: There are three basic treatments for allergy: avoidance, medication, and allergy injections. Cortisone, which is a steroid, is a fourth choice because it can cause serious side effects.

Helpful hint 2: Allergy injections do not have to be taken forever, especially if you are willing to go along with the high dose method of treatment.

Helpful hint 3: Work cooperatively with your allergist. Be ready to tell him which of the possible treatments fits your situation, which ones you are willing to follow, and which ones you are reluctant to follow. This will help him help *you*.

Why Allergy Symptoms Are Often Worse At Night

Many allergy patients feel worse at night. When Dr. Michael Smolensky at the University of Texas tried to find out the reason, he couldn't discover a *single* factor that explained all cases.

Some people are worse due to more intense exposure to household allergens, such as dust, pets, and feathers, which they are exposed to throughout the evening while they are at home.

In others the protective level of an adrenal hormone drops during the night and allows allergy symptoms to surface. Certain adrenal hormones decrease at night in everyone, but when this happens in an allergic patient the decrease can trigger allergy symptoms. The effect is so common that some people mistakenly conclude that adrenal hormone deficiency *causes* allergy in the first place. Although this idea is intriguing, it has been proven false.

A third contributing factor to nighttime symptoms is an increase in reactivity of the lung's airways that occurs in some patients.

Thus, those of you who are worse at night must consult your doctors and investigate your *particular* reason for nighttime symptoms. Only by doing this can you learn how to control your allergies effectively.

> **Helpful hint 1**: If your allergies are worse at night, you should ask your doctor to help you figure out why. This will help you control your symptoms better than if you and your doctor try to *guess* why you are worse at night.

> **Helpful hint 2**: If your allergies are worse at night, consider adjusting the time at which you take your medicine so it coincides with and prevents your increased symptoms.

> **Helpful hint 3**: In allergy, as in other medical specialties, there are often several explanations for a particular problem. This is why it is important to see a physician who specializes. She will be familiar with all the different possibilities and help you figure out which one is the one that is causing your particular problem.

More Reasons Why You Need To See A Specialist

Dr. Wantke Hemmer who is a doctor in Vienna did an interesting study which shows how important it is to see a specialist.

Dr. Hemmer studied a woman who had asthma after drinking red wine. This patient had already been proven allergic to certain pollens that caused her to have hayfever.

So, here was a patient who was known to be allergic to ordinary pollens and was suddenly reacting to wine.

Dr. Hemmer resisted the temptation to simply label this patient as wine-allergic. Instead the doctor took the trouble to investigate the problem and found that this woman was reacting to the histamine in wine because her body lacked an enzyme, called diamine oxidase, that metabolizes the histamine in wine so it doesn't harm us. This allows the rest of us to drink as much wine as we want. Well, not *too* much. And *none* if you're going to drive.

Helpful hint 1: Without thorough knowledge of the ins and outs of allergy, it can be tempting to label any adverse reaction an allergy. This can lead to a faulty diagnosis and a faulty treatment.

Helpful hint 2: Whether you react to wine or not, do not drink alcohol and drive.

Discovery Of The Worst Location For Allergy

After a short time in practice, I realized that many allergic individuals believe the only reason they are ill with allergy is that they are unlucky enough to be living in the "worst area of the country" for allergy. This is never correct because there is not a worst area of the country for allergy.

In the United States the incidence of *susceptibility* to allergy is pretty steady at about 30 percent of the population. In fact, this percentage is similar throughout the world. But susceptibility just means you have the *potential* for developing symptoms. Unless you are exposed to *your* allergens, you won't feel a thing. For example, if you are violently allergic to peanuts but never eat them, you will not be ill. Or if you have asthma due to trees and move to an area which has only grass, you won't have asthma. Of course if you move to tree-country, you will cough and wheeze. You will feel awful. And if you are like most people, you will conclude that you have just moved to the worst part of the country for allergy.

What do you think a person would say about the worst place for allergy if they were allergic to cats and brought their cats with them when they moved? In this situation, *everyplace* is the worst.

Thus, allergy symptoms do not depend on a specific state, country, or continent. They depend on what you are allergic to *and* how much you are exposed to the substances to which you are allergic.

However, I can now disclose, and this may surprise you, that the area of the United States with the highest percentage of allergy is Arizona. Surprised?

Years ago allergy sufferers moved to desert areas like Arizona to escape exposure to pollens. There, they intermarried and had children. Since the ability to make excess IgE antibody, which is the root-cause of allergy, is an inherited characteristic, most of their children wound up with this gene and made excess IgE. In fact, when allergy sufferer married allergy sufferer, they gave their children a double dose of susceptibility, a dose from each parent.

Then, thanks to irrigation, these allergy sufferers planted trees and grasses. And wouldn't you know it, they planted the very trees and grasses they were trying to avoid in the first place. They also brought their pets. They created dust. Eventually the citizens of Arizona had an environment full of allergenic substances. With so many predisposed people waiting to make IgE antibody, you can guess what happened. Arizona wound up with more allergic individuals than other states.

Helpful hint 1: The worst area in the United States is different for different people. This depends on what you are sensitive to *and* what allergens are in your environment.

Helpful hint 2: Because allergy is inherited and because years ago people with allergies moved to Arizona, intermarried, and had children, Arizona now has the highest percentage of allergic individuals in the United States.

Helpful hint 3: If you want to move someplace and a friend tells you it is the worst place for allergies, it may be the worst place for your friend, but this does not mean it will be the worst place for you.

Discovery Of The Worst Year For Allergy Sufferers

When I began practicing allergy, local newspapers and radio stations routinely called me during the height of the allergy season to ask if this was the worst year I had encountered. I understood their interest because Silicon Valley (Santa Clara County) has a reputation for being the worst area in the country for allergy sufferers. If a reporter could put the worst year together with the worst area, that reporter would have one darn good headline.

I responded to such questions with a complicated answer where I explained about pollen counts, wind factors, availability of medication, and the subjective feelings of patients. I'm sure it sounded like double-talk. As a result, the journalists stopped calling me.

Nevertheless, every year I read a headline which states, "Worst Year Ever According to Dr. So and So."

When I see such a headline, I have this urge to cut it out and send it to the newspaper the following year with the question, "How can you print this again? How can every year be the worst year? One year has to be the *second* worst year."

On the other hand, "second worst years" don't sell newspapers.

A few facts which do not seem to interest reporters will explain how you judge the severity of a year. One factor is the actual pollen count. The more pollen in the air, the worse the year. Second in importance is the *strength* of the pollen. Depending on the previous year's growing conditions, various plant pollens will be weaker or stronger. A barrelful of inactive pollen (inactive in allergic terms) cannot compare to a cupful of highly potent pollen. Third, the wind, rain, barometric pressure and smog level can increase or decrease the severity of allergy symptoms.

Thus, there are *multiple* factors involved in determining how bad a year is. Focusing on only one factor is bound to be misleading. And trying to assess the severity of a season in the *middle* of a season *before all the facts are in* is impossible. What if it suddenly starts raining and washes all the pollen away?

The only way to know if a particular year is the worst year in history is to wait until the season ends, count how many people saw allergists compared to previous years, add up the number of prescriptions sold that year, and count the amount of Kleenex people used.

Even if allergists seem extraordinarily busy and have patients falling out the windows when the newspaper reporter calls, there could be a sudden change in the weather. The season could end abruptly two days later. However, waiting for the truth to make itself known is not something newspaper and radio reporters know how to do.

Helpful hint 1: There are many factors that influence how severe a particular allergy season will be.

Helpful hint 2: You cannot tell which is the worst year ever unless you wait until the season ends, count the number of allergy visits during the season, and compare the total to previous seasons. No one bothers to collect this information.

Helpful hint 3: The true facts of a situation are often not newsworthy.

2

Newly Discovered
Allergens
and
Chemical Mediators

If you think medical science knows all the possible substances that can cause allergy because we already know about dogs, cats, ragweed, and dust, you are wrong. There are still new allergens to be discovered. It is important to learn about new allergens because if a patient says he is reacting to a particular substance, we doctors don't want to dismiss the story because scientists hadn't known this substance was allergenic. The following studies tell you about substances that you wouldn't usually suspect as being able to cause an allergic reaction. One is a vitamin. The other is a healthy, natural food. The third study explains how hi-tech gene research is helping us characterize the specific molecules in each and every allergen.

The second part of this chapter tells you what we have learned about the process whereby allergens cause symptoms. You need three ingredients, sort of a witches' brew. You need IgE antibody, an allergen such as grass pollen, food, animal dander, or dust, and a chemical your body produces called a mediator. Chemical mediators are chemicals that your body produces *internally*. Without them, dogs, cats, dust, and ragweed cannot affect you. Chemical mediators are the go-between that translates the IgE-allergen reaction into actual symptoms in your nose, eyes, lungs, skin, and sinuses. Chemical mediators are the substances that make you feel ill. So to treat allergy better, allergists spend a lot of time studying chemical mediators.

The most well-known chemical mediator is histamine. You make histamine in your Mast cells which are one of hundreds of cells in your body. To block histamine, you take an *anti*-histamine. I wish all allergy was as simple as this. Unfortunately, there are many other chemical mediators that can make you as sick as histamine can....or worse! And we do not yet have good antidotes for many of the other mediators. Scientists who work for drug companies are in a race to learn as much as they can about the other chemical mediators so their respective companies can make an antidote. The last study in this section tells you about this. The winning drug company will earn our thanks, sell a lot of pills, and make a lot of money.

Discovery That Vitamins Can Cause Allergic Reactions

Vitamins are supposed to be beneficial and harmless. So when Dr. Jerry Dolovich from Canada found a man who collapsed and had seizures after taking a vitamin C tablet, allergists stood up and paid attention. The man had such a severe reaction he wound up in an intensive care unit.

After a great deal of investigation, Dr. Dolovich and his co-workers discovered the culprit. This was polyethylene glycol, a chemical which bound the various ingredients in the vitamin C tablet. Polyethylene glycol is used in many medicinal tablets besides vitamin C.

This shows you that you never know how or where allergy will strike. Even something as harmless as a vitamin can cause a severe reaction.

Helpful hint 1: Allergy reactions can occur in the most unexpected circumstances, so always monitor your body and report any adverse reactions to your doctor right away.

Helpful hint 2: Many people think they are allergic to various drugs when in fact they are not allergic to the active ingredient but to one of the other substances used to make the tablet.

Helpful hint 3: Just for fun, I thought you might be interested in seeing a list of various ingredients commonly used to manufacture tablets. It is astounding to learn that when you purchase a drug for its active ingredient, you get a whole bunch of other substances too.

• Filler-- an ingredient that fills tablets or capsules (e.g. dicalcium phosphate, vegetable oil).
• Binder-- a substance that holds tablets together (e.g. lactose, cornstarch).
• Lubricant-- a chemical that allows tablets to be ejected from the compression mold (e.g. magnesium stearate).
• Glidant-- an ingredient that prevents blended material from clumping (e.g. a mineral from hydrated silica).
• Disintegrant-- a substance that makes tablets break apart in the digestive tract (e.g. starch).
• Coating-- a chemical that protects tablets from light or moisture (e.g. sugar).
• Flavor and Sweetener-- substances that are found in chewable and liquid drugs (e.g. fructose, sorbitol).

• Color-- a chemical used for identification. This can be natural or artificial (e.g. carotene, tartrazine).

Helpful hint 4: Vitamins can be harmful to your health.

Natural Healthy Carrots Cause Allergy

Dr. Samuel Lehrer from New Orleans treated a patient who developed swelling of the throat and difficulty breathing within minutes after eating a carrot. Since carrots are supposed to be healthy and full of vitamins, this was hard to believe. But on subsequent testing the person reacted each time, thus proving that carrots can be healthy for some and nearly deadly for others.

Helpful hint 1: Even natural, healthy foods are bad for you if you are allergic to them.

How Smog Causes Allergy

While Dr. Michael Glovsky and his colleagues were studying allergy in Los Angeles, which is sometimes dubbed the smog capital of the United States, among other unflattering epithets, he and his coworkers learned that 10,000 pounds of rubber tire particles are released into the air each day. Performing sophisticated studies, the doctors found that latex, a natural constituent of the rubber in tires, was present in these particles.

In a separate study using a special test that measures IgE antibody for latex, the doctors found that many asthmatic patients had high levels of IgE latex-antibody which indicated that the patients were likely susceptible to latex.

With these two findings in mind the doctors proposed that latex from tires is one of the factors that contributes to increased allergic asthma on smoggy days. They are continuing their studies to prove this one way or the other.

Helpful hint 1: Regardless of whether it proves to be latex or one of the other constituents of dirty air such as nitrous oxide, carbon particles, or dirt that exacerbates allergies, you need to take extra precautions on smoggy days.

A Bodily Chemical Is Found To Be Responsible For Allergic Reactions
(Or, The Real Story Why Antihistamines Don't Always Work.)

After hearing so much about IgE causing allergy, you may feel cheated to learn that I only told you half the story about what causes allergy. You also need *chemical mediators*. These are naturally-made chemicals that your body produces. All of us make these chemicals, not just allergic people. They are important in maintaining bodily function, repairing tissue, repelling infection, and keeping us healthy.

On the one hand I've told you chemical mediators make you ill with allergy. On the other hand I've said they are necessary to maintain your health. So what is the truth?

Chemical mediators are made and stored in various cells in the body. Ordinarily they are released in small amounts when they are required for normal, physiologic function. However, if you have too much IgE antibody, your body loses control of the way it releases certain of its chemical mediators. Like many chemicals in the body such as thyroid, insulin, calcium, and so forth, *too much* or *inappropriate release when not needed* will cause symptoms. In the case of allergy it is the inappropriate release triggered by too much IgE antibody that is the problem.

The most well known chemical mediator is histamine. Patients often ask if they are allergic because they have too much histamine in their body. Strictly speaking, if you are allergic you are not *overflowing* with histamine. Your cells contain just the normal amount. However, when your cells release the histamine at inappropriate times, you will have symptoms.

> *It is not too much histamine but rather the inappropriate release of histamine that causes allergy symptoms.*

Other Bodily Chemicals That Contribute To Allergy

Below is a list of other chemicals your body makes and needs for its normal function but which under certain circumstances cause allergy symptoms. Like histamine, they can be inappropriately released. When this occurs, they can provoke symptoms. Dr. Frank Austen, who has done a lot of research in this area, is an articulate lecturer on this subject. Many laboratories throughout the world are trying to develop antidotes for each of these mediators. If they are successful, they will be financially rewarded. Your reward will be feeling better.

Bradykinin
Growth Colony Factors
HETE
Histamine
Histamine Releasing Factors
Interferon

Interleukin
Kinin
Leukotriene
Lysyl Bradykinin
Major Basic Protein
Nitrous Oxide
PAF (platelet activating factor)
PGD
Prostaglandin
SRS-A
TAME esterase activity
Thromboxane
Tryptase

Although these names are long, difficult to pronounce, and probably boring to you, they are exciting to allergists. If we can learn which chemical mediator is responsible for a particular symptom and if the drug companies can discover a safe antidote, just like *anti*histamine is the antidote for histamine, we will be able to help you better.

Many times I've wished histamine was the only chemical mediator we had to deal with because we already have its antidote. Unfortunately, the other chemicals on the list are responsible for just as many allergic reactions as histamine. This explains why antihistamines alone don't always help you.

Misleading Reports About Allergy Cures

When it comes to believing what you read in newspapers and magazines about medical breakthroughs, you must be cautious. Certain newspaper reporters don't have the technical expertise to evaluate medical information. They frequently rely on a person who is enthusiastic but biased about a particular research study's findings. In the field of allergy, chemical mediators are sometimes subject to this kind of twisted reporting.

Over the years I've read many feature stories that make me think a miraculous cure is just around the corner. In their zeal to create eye-catching headlines, some reporters ignore the words of cautious doctors who explain that a particular discovery is a *preliminary* finding.

Since allergy researchers are constantly finding chemical mediators, there is always something new. So far, though, no one has found a particular chemical mediator that, by itself, is *solely* responsible for every type of allergic condition. The dominant chemical mediator that causes sneezing in one individual is often different from the one that causes sneezing in another individual. To make matters more complicated, it is usually a *combination* of chemical mediators that causes sneezing in a particular individual. The kind of wishy-washy news report that says the answer is different for different people doesn't make a good headline. It's better to print, "New, Micracle, and Cure" than "Doctors have found another link in the chain".

Even when doctors isolate chemical mediators and demonstrate which ones are responsible for allergic reactions, the doctors still have to invent drugs to counteract the mediators. Even if they could do that, they would then need to test the drugs for safety in children, adults, and pregnant women. Then they would have to figure out which drug works for a particular individual without producing serious side effects.

At this stage of my medical career, it is too much for me to believe that doctors will soon have a single, magic pill that works for everyone.

Additionally, none of the mediators on the above list are *truly* new, unless in your mind "new" covers the last five to ten years. The mediators that have captured the media's fancy are interleukins, leukotrienes, TAME esterase activity, and Histamine Releasing Factors.

The antidotes for some of these mediators have been identified and manufactured. For example, antidotes to prostaglandins are Zileuton, Rolipram, and Siguazodan, to leukotriene are Interferon Gamma and Zafirlukast (Acolate), to eosinophils and Major Basic Protein is Humanized Anti-IL-5 antibodies. After years studying these so-called new mediators and their antidotes, though, the final verdict isn't in. So, I'm sorry to say this, but when you read of the next latest breakthrough in finding "the cause" of allergy, don't get your hopes too high.

Helpful hint 1: Several normal chemicals made by the human body participate in causing allergic reactions. Although these chemicals are important for your everyday physiologic function, the cells of allergic patients, in combination with excess IgE antibody, release these chemicals inappropriately. This is what causes allergy symptoms.

Helpful hint 2: There have been no truly new chemicals discovered in many years. But doctors are learning new things about the ones that have already been found.

Helpful hint 3: Hopefully, understanding the many interactions between chemical mediators, IgE, and allergens such as dog dander, dust, and pollens, will enable your doctors to control your allergies better.

Helpful hint 4: For a reason unkown to me, when doctors discover new drugs, they make up names, like Zafirlukast and Siguazodan, that are nearly impossible to pronounce.

3

Allergy Testing

Before you start allergy treatment, you must have proof that your symptoms are due to allergy. Many diseases mimic allergy such as infection, enzyme deficiency, irritant chemicals, food intolerance, and structural abnormalities in the nose and sinuses, to name just a few. If you suffer from an allergy-mimic, allergy treatment would be of no use. You would be off in the wrong direction before you got started.

The bottom line is this: If you or your doctor think you have allergy, you need an evaluation. An essential part of an allergy evaluation is allergy testing. Testing verifies what you are allergic to. Well-meaning friends, your intuition, and even doctors may try to tell you what you are allergic to. However, without confirmatory proof from specific tests their opinion is nothing more than an opinion. Maybe they're right, and maybe they aren't. They have nothing to lose by guessing. You do.

Tests come in all shapes, sizes, and forms. There are prick, scratch, intradermal, blood, provocation, sublingual, muscle, and diet tests. It will be helpful for you to know more about these tests. This is what this chapter is about. Also, you should re-read *Will The Real Allergist Please Stand Up* to refresh your memory about who does what kind of test.

Allergy testing can be simple and quick, or it can be complex, costly, and time-consuming. The method utilized depends on your doctor's training and sometimes on *your* expectations. Some doctors don't have the time to study the various tests and may not appreciate the benefits and disadvantages of each type. On the other hand, you may believe you get what you pay for and think that the more tests done and the more expensive they are, the better the doctor.

In actual practice, you can be tested in fifteen minutes for every allergen imaginable. And the results are available immediately.

The first of the following studies explains what we have learned about the grouping method of testing. This technique reduces the total number of tests needed to investigate airborne allergens and still disclose all the significant information. The second study explains how doctors proved that most food allergy tests are only twenty percent accurate. The last study explains all you need to know (and perhaps more than you want to know) about the three commonly-used blood tests for diagnosing food allergy.

How To Reduce The Number Of Allergy Tests For Airborne Allergens
(Or, How To Cut The Cost Of An Allergy Workup)

Allergists don't want to make the mistake of overlooking an allergen that might be contributing to your symptoms. So certain doctors run 100, 150, or even 200 tests. Although this will sound like a contradiction, doctors can learn the same information from seventy-five tests as from 200 tests.

When it comes to airborne allergens such as grasses, trees, and weeds, certain plants belong in families. If you are allergic to one member of a family of plants, you are allergic to the other members of the same family. For example, it is unnecessary to test you for red, yellow, pink, and white roses. A single test for the basic rose plant provides the same information as multiple tests for each variety of rose. People who are allergic to roses are not allergic to the color. They are allergic to the plant itself.

There was recent proof of this from the laboratory of Dr. Jean Bousquet in France. Dr. Bousquet showed that members of the Oleacea family (olive, ash, privet, and phillyrea) contain the same allergen. Thus, a person who is allergic to olive is allergic to the other three species as well.

I have mixed emotions when I explain this grouping method of testing. It's like having to apologize for being practical. But many patients equate the number of tests their doctor performs to the thoroughness of their allergy workup. They mistakenly believe that the more tests done the better their evaluation.

Another way to reduce the number of tests is to omit tests for such things as camels and goats, unless, of course, you live with a camel or a goat. The principle behind omitting tests for camels and goats is this: If you are not exposed to an allergen, the allergen cannot affect you no matter how allergic you are. To cite two practical examples, if you are highly allergic to kangaroos, you will never be bothered unless you live in a zoo. If you are fatally allergic to peanuts, you cannot have symptoms unless you eat peanuts.

Helpful hint 1: It is rare that you require more than seventy-five scratch tests for a complete allergic analysis.

Helpful hint 2: An allergy workup is less costly and time consuming when fewer tests are done, yet the workup can still be thorough *if* the tests are chosen properly.

Inaccuracy Of Food Tests Confirmed

Food allergy is baffling to many people. Although there is no doubt that food allergy exists, there is a great deal of confusion over what types of problems food allergy can cause and how to investigate food allergy.

Two Types Of Hidden Food Allergy

There are two types of hidden food allergy. The first is *immediate*. This occurs within a few minutes after you eat a food. The second is *delayed*. This occurs hours to days *after* you eat the food because foods must be digested, absorbed, converted to energy, and the unuseable by-products must be eliminated. We call this metabolism. Along the way various food byproducts are created. These byproducts, rather than the food itself, cause delayed reactions.

People who react to *unmetabolized* foods are *immediate* reactors. People who react to *metabolized* foods are *delayed* reactors.

Immediate reactions to unmetabolized foods typically cause hives, itching, facial and tongue swelling, asthma, difficulty breathing, and in some cases death. Delayed reactions to metabolized foods cause numerous kinds of symptoms such as headaches, asthma, fatigue, and nasal symptoms, to name a few.

The Problem With Blood And Skin Tests For Food Allergy

The primary roadblock to successful food-allergy testing is the lack of appropriate allergens. Doctors would need unmetabolized and metabolized forms of *every* food you eat so they could test you for immediate and delayed reactions. This is shown in the following table.

Type of Reaction	Immediate	Delayed
Food responsible	Natural, unmetabolized and undigested	Metabolized and digested
Availability for testing	Available	Unavailable

In the United States, we do not have metabolized foods for testing. They are unstable. Even if they were stable, there are dozens of breakdown products for each food. This is because the digestive process is long and involved. So doctors have no choice but to use natural (undigested) foods for skin and blood tests. Yet this only uncovers *immediate*-type food reactions which are the obvious ones. Immediate reactions begin within minutes after you ingest the food. You know that something is wrong right away. You do not usually need a doctor to tell you.

The delayed reactions, which are due to metabolized by-products, are the ones that are difficult to pinpoint because they can occur from hours to days later. Delayed reactions are the ones that we need help uncovering. Unfortunately, as I said above, delayed reactions are the ones for which test-allergens are not available.

The more you study food allergy, the more complicated it becomes. Not only do you have to consider metabolized and unmetabolized foods, you also have to consider *combinations* of foods. You need to consider whether a food is cooked or uncooked, too. In the early 1900's Dr. Otto Prausnitz, who is considered one of the founders of modern allergy research, showed that a person can be allergic to cooked but not to raw egg. The person he used as a guinea pig was Heinz Kustner, who later went on to become an obstetrician. I suppose Dr. Kustner's first brush with food allergy research in Dr. Prausnitz's lab convinced him he should do anything to avoid the allergy field! He must have wanted to do something easy like delivering babies.

In a more recent study that is reminiscent of Dr. Prausnitz's work, Dr. James Rosen warned allergists that they need to test with raw and cooked food or they would risk making a mistake. You need to use the exact form of the food that caused the reaction. For example, you cannot use apple juice to test a person who thinks they react to apple sauce. You can't test a person with raw carrot, if they reacted to cooked carrot. If you are testing for raw carrot, you may need to leave the skin on. Or you may need to expose the carrot to air for awhile because the problem could be due to an oxidized coating on the carrot from exposure to air. I could go on and on like this, but you get the point.

In fact, Dr. Hong Oei of the Netherlands microwaved an apple and fed it to an apple-allergic patient. This converted the apple to a non-allergenic food *for that particular patient*. So you can see how a slight modification changes a food from allergenic to non-allergenic, and visa versa.

Despite what I've just said, some patients still want to believe that skin and blood tests, even using imperfect allergens, will help them uncover their food allergies. They are willing to suspend logic and ignore scientific fact in the hope that they can avoid an *elimination diet*, where, as the name implies, they must stop eating certain foods to see if their symptoms go away, and a *provocative challenge* diet, where they eat the food to see if their symptoms begin. Unfortunately these two food tests are the only one-hundred percent accurate food-tests now available to us.

If you still have faith in skin and blood food tests after reading the above, Dr. Charles Reed of the Mayo Clinic will spoil your faith. He has figured out *exactly* how inaccurate skin and blood tests are. Talk about giving allergists and patients a serving of humility when it comes to food allergy, Dr. Reed has given us a big portion.

He performed skin and blood test on 102 people who told him they had food allergy. The tests were abnormal in thirty-one of the 102 individuals.

Dr. Reed went on to double-check whether the tests were accurate using a tried and true method. He fed the supposedly allergenic food to the supposedly allergic thirty-one people. If they had been *truly* allergic, they would have reacted upon eating the food. This is the *provocative challenge* test I mentioned above. Not wanting his subjects to be influenced by knowing what they were eating, Dr. Reed put the foods in capsules and liquids to disguise the flavor and taste.

Of the thirty-one people who had positive tests, seven reacted upon eating the food. So, of the original 102 who thought they were allergic, only thirty-one had positive skin or blood tests. Of these only seven had symptoms upon eating the food. This translates to an accuracy of twenty-one percent (7/31). This is not good! Twenty-one percent accurate means seventy-nine percent *inaccurate*.

Helpful hint 1: Anyone who advocates relying on a test that is accurate only twenty-one percent of the time has got to be kidding! If you flip a coin, you get fifty percent accuracy.

Helpful hint 2: Anyone who lets himself be talked into doing a test that is accurate twenty-one percent of the time is desperate and grasping at straws.

Helpful hint 3: Twenty-one percent accuracy is true for the four skin tests, three blood tests, and the under-the-tongue (sublingual) tests that are in use today (see below).

Helpful hint 4: When it comes to subjecting patients to food tests, you can fool a lot of people by advocating high-tech medicine like blood tests or professing faith in old-fashioned medicine like sublingual drop tests.

Helpful hint 5: The best test for food allergy is a double-blind, placebo-controlled, food challenge.

Three Blood Tests For Food Allergy

There are three types of blood test for food allergy; cytotoxic, histamine release, and RAST. All blood tests are variations of these three. However because there is a high profit margin in blood tests various companies have created many variations. They hope a gullible public will spend its money on hopes and dreams because medical science cannot provide an easy answer. The last time I counted there were over eight variations of the three basic food tests.

Cytotoxic Test (Bryan's test, FICA test, Food Immune Complex Assay)

In the cytotoxic test, doctors separate your white from your red blood cells, add a food or chemical, and observe whether the cells break apart. If the cells break, you are said to be allergic to the food.

Regrettably, the cytotoxic test has been proven highly inaccurate. The substances that are used for cytotoxic testing are *unmetabolized* instead of metabolized foods. Furthermore, many things kill your white cells. Simply removing them from the protected environment of your body kills them.

The cytotoxic test was developed in the early 1950's by a Dr. Bryan (hence the original name Bryan's test). Thorough investigation has repeatedly shown the test is inconsistent.

One day an unmetabolized food kills cells. Another day the same food doesn't kill the cells. Furthermore, this test does not take into account the effect of combinations of foods or whether a food is cooked, uncooked, pasteurized, frozen, microwaved, or otherwise processed in a way that alters the food. Medical schools, university laboratories, and licensed laboratories don't perform cytotoxic tests. Trained allergists don't do them. Only certain physicians do them in the privacy of their office.

The doctors who advocate cytotoxic tests claim the test can discover the cause of cancer, weight problems, emotional disturbances, headaches, arthritis, gynecologic problems, and other diseases too numerous to mention.

> *If cytotoxic tests were helpful for half as many diseases as claimed, all your medical conditions would be due to allergy and the only physician you would need throughout your life would be an allergist.*

Histamine Release Test

The histamine release test is similar to the cytotoxic test in the respect that doctors use your white blood cells and add foods and pollens for stimulation.

However instead of examining your cells for breakage, they measure the amount of histamine your cells release. Instead of examining your leukocyte-type white cells as is done in the cytotoxic test, they examine basophil-type white cells.

The histamine test is accurate when used for pollens. However, when used for foods, the histamine test is as inaccurate as the cytotoxic test for the same reason-- *unmetabolized* foods are used instead of *metabolized by-*

products. Additionally the test makes no distinction between cooked, uncooked, microwaved, boiled, pasteurized, unpasteurized, or combinations of foods.

RAST Test

Finally there is the RAST-family of tests which go under the names RAST, FAST, PRIST, ELISA, MAST, RIST, STALLERZYM, and CAP. Like skin tests, RAST tests measure IgE antibody.

For airborne allergens, RAST-type tests are almost as accurate as skin tests. However, for *food* allergy RAST-type tests are inaccurate because they utilize *unmetabolized* foods instead of *metabolized, digested by-products* and they do not take into account cooked, uncooked, microwaved, boiled, pasteurized, unpasteurized, or combinations of foods.

In addition to being less accurate, RAST-type tests cost four to five times more than skin tests.

The *Accurate* Food Allergy Test

My remarks may make you feel hopeless about detecting food allergy. But, don't despair! There's a test that is 100 percent accurate, *always* works, and is cheap! It is the elimination-diet test. If you stop eating a food and get better and eat the food and reproduce your symptoms, this food is making you sick and you should stop eating it.

Helpful hint 1: There are no new blood tests for food allergy. There are only aggressive companies trying to market new versions of blood tests that are fifteen to thirty years old. By the time you read this book, you will undoubtedly hear of other "new" tests as marketing people become more inventive with new names for the old tests.

Helpful hint 2: Blood tests cost four to five times more than skin tests.

Helpful hint 3: Because airborne allergens don't have to be metabolized by the body into an allergenic form, blood and skin tests for *airborne* allergens are *accurate*. On the other hand, because food allergens often need to be metabolized into their allergenic form, blood and skin tests for *food* allergens are *inaccurate*.

Helpful hint 4: Blood and skin tests for foods can lead to a common medical mistake which is to ignore *you* and treat your tests.

Helpful hint 5: To convince you to pay for costly blood tests, certain health care professionals cast aspersions on *skin* tests by saying that skin tests are not accurate because they do not account for delays in reactions or for combinations of foods. They also remind you how tedious it is to stick to an elimination diet.

These people are correct! There can be delays in onset of symptoms due to foods, food reactions can be due to combinations of foods, skin tests are inaccurate, and elimination diets are tedious. But, and this is a big but, blood tests are no better. In fact they are worse! Because they seem modern, new, and technical, they give you false hopes and make you think you can buy your answers without any effort on your part.

Helpful hint 6: If you insist on obtaining blood or skin tests to detect possible food allergies, you are looking for an easy way out. You are responding to advertising claims that reinforce what you want to hear instead of what is true.

Helpful hint 7: There is only one test that is 100 percent accurate for food allergy. This test is an elimination diet. If total abstinence from a food corrects your problem, the food causes the problem. Otherwise, something else is responsible for your symptoms.

4

House Dust Control and The Home Environment

Allergy to house dust is one of the most common allergies in existence because house dust is everywhere and you are exposed to it from the day you are born. Contrary to what you may think, however, the dust that causes allergic problems is not the same as the dirt you find on the ground. Allergic-type dust comes from plant by-products such as cotton and kapok and from insects such as house dust mite and cockroaches. Allergenic house dust does not include dirt, pebbles, cookie crumbs, and other inert matter found on the floors of most of our homes. Nor does it include animal dander and mold spores. These allergens are distinct and have their own chapters in this book.

So when you think of house dust you must think from an allergist's point of view. Think cotton and kapok stuffing-material, house dust mite, and cockroaches.

The following studies illuminate little-known facts about the best methods to control allergy to house dust and house dust mites, the effectiveness of air purifiers, air conditioners, humidifiers, and ionizers, problems that have been reported due to home insulation, how allergy to dust mites may really be due to allergy to cats, and finally the best way to vacuum your home.

House Dust Mite Allergy

House dust mites are microscopic insects that live in rugs and in the cotton and kapok stuffing-material used in mattresses, boxsprings, pillows, and chairs. Allergists love to show you a greatly magnified picture of a dust mite (Dermatophagoides Pteronyssinus) because the insects look so scary. They produce material which can enter the air you breathe and provoke allergy if you are susceptible.

Dr. S. T. Roeseler from Dusseldorf, Germany listed the known varieties of mites in a study he did on the occurrence of mites in Europe. To give you an idea of how many types there are, I've listed them too.

Pteronyssinus, Farinae, Euroglyphus Maynei, Tyrophagus Putrescentiae, Acarus Siro, Glycyphagus Domesticus, Lepidoglyphyus Destructor. (I can't pronounce these names any better than you can.)

Dr. M. Chapman, PhD, from Manchester, England, has developed a rapid test to detect mites in the home. As is usual in scientific research these days, he used a genetic engineering technique and never did say how much this would cost. But at least someone is working on a way for us to know what we're dealing with in cases of mite allergy.

Of course, even if you don't detect mites in your home this doesn't mean they are never there. You may have missed their season. Or you may have tested in the wrong place. So if you are allergic to mites it is best to *assume* they are there and take the precautions that are described below. These are based on the experiences of many doctors who have studied how to control allergy to mites and prevent allergic reactions from these insects.

First, the most successful method is an old, tried-and-true, and favorite technique of allergists everywhere. Encase your mattress, boxspring, and pillows inside specially designed mattress encasings. In addition, you may do any of the following.

Dr. Platts-Mills reported that he was able to rid a house of dust mites using a chemical called primiphos methyl. A single treatment lasted up to six weeks. Benzyl benzoate and tannic acid have also helped to varying degrees. Dr. Richard Lockey showed that caffeine, like the caffeine in coffee, is another chemical that can effectively lower the concentration of mites in your home. Dr. Euan Tovey showed that exposing a carpet to the heat of direct sunlight for about six hours kills mites. Dr. G. David Hopper showed that killing mites isn't enough. After using chemicals to kill mites, you need to vacuum their remains. Otherwise, their debris, such as dead mites and mite-droppings, circulate and cause symptoms.

Another well-known way to reduce the mite population is to maintain the humidity below fifty percent. Mites don't breed well in low humidity. The fewer the mites, the fewer the symptoms they can trigger in you.

J. Dippold from Dayton, Ohio, studied how to kill mites with heat. This is useful to know for washing your blankets and sheets. Washing at 70 degrees Celsius (158 Farenheit) killed mites in thirty minutes. At 60 degrees Celsius (140 degrees Farenheit) it took one and a half hours.

Finally, many doctors recommend a program of immunizing allergy injections to build your resistance to mites.

Whichever way you choose to control mites, you must keep doing it. Mites are relentless little buggers (sorry for the pun) and you need to keep after them to eliminate them from your environment.

Helpful hint 1: House dust mites can provoke allergic symptoms in susceptible individuals.

Helpful hint 2: Even if a skin test shows you are super-allergic to dust mites, you will not experience symptoms unless there are mites in your environment. So in parts of the United States where the lack of humidity prevents mites from growing, you don't have to worry about positive skin tests to mites since there would be few mites to bother you.

Helpful hint 3: As is true with most allergenic substances, there are various ways of coping. With dust mite allergy, you can buy mattress encasings, lower the humidity, use chemicals to kill them, or get allergy immunizing injections.

Helpful hint 4: If you use a chemical to kill insects such as dust mites, be careful that you do not react to the chemical itself.

Helpful hint 5: If you are allergic to house dust mite but mite allergy is a small part of your total problem, you are better off spending your time and energy taking care of the other allergens first.

Helpful hint 6: If you do not want to use chemicals with strange names to kill mites, you can spill coffee, which contains caffeine, on your rug (only joking!).

Dust-Proof The Home in One Easy Step

The greatest sources of cotton and kapok stuffing and dust mite allergens are mattresses, boxsprings, and pillows. Studies show that thousands of mites live in happy contentment in the stuffing material that is used to make mattresses and boxsprings. It probably sounds disgusting to hear that these creatures are swarming in your bed at a concentration of hundreds to the inch, but you would probably also be disgusted to learn how many bacteria live on your skin, in your mouth, and deep in your gastrointestinal tract. I won't even give you the numbers.

There are sprays, liquids, powders, washing techniques, and various ways you can condition your home to reduce the mite population, but my favorite way is to bury them. This is a one-step procedure and has proven to be highly effective.

Purchase special encasings from any of the numerous companies that sell them. The only scientific requirement is that the material must be impermeable to water. If water cannot get through, nothing can get through. Put your mattress, boxspring, and pillows inside the encasing, zip up, and seal with tape. You have now isolated the mites in their own little world and need not worry about them bothering you again.

Helpful hint 1: In allergy, avoidance is the best policy.

Helpful hint 2: Allergy encasings are an allergist's best friend for treating house-dust allergy. If you use an encasing, the encasing will be your best friend, too.

Effectiveness Of Air Cleaners

There are two types machines that clean the air for dust-sensitive patients. They both contain a fan to blow air through a special cleansing unit. One machine cleans the air with a sponge-like material called High Efficiency Particle Absorbent (HEPA). The other machine contains two electrified metal plates. As air passes between the plates, the electric charge attracts and holds small particles. This is called electrostatic cleaning.

According to environmental engineers, both types of machine successfully clean the air. But allergists are not interested in cleaning the air. They are interested in getting you better. You would think cleaning the air and making you feel better would be the same. It turns out they are not.

Upon investigation of homes with air cleaners, Dr. Charles Reed found shelves were cleaner, floors looked better, and patients had to do a lot less dusting. But only one-fourth of the patients improved. Needless to say, this was very disappointing to Dr. Reed.

This outcome is surprising until you think about it. There are several reasons for the lack of improvement despite having clean air.

• Filters clog when you run an air cleaner continuously.

• Most people are allergic to outdoor substances, too.

• You can't isolate yourself in your house all day since you can't conduct your life in a bubble.

• The blowers that circulate the air through these machines also circulate allergens which might otherwise lie on the ground and not bother you.

Helpful hint 1: Although air cleaners can do a wonderful job of cleaning your home, they won't necessarily relieve your allergy symptoms.

Helpful hint 2: Since air cleaners are not guaranteed to help you, you should use them on a trial basis to see if they are worth purchasing.

Helpful hint 3: People ought to know better than to expect much help from a treatment that is designed for dust allergy but does nothing for other allergens such as pollens and food.

Helpful hint 4: Air conditioners cool the air, humidifiers moisten the air, and ionizers put ions into the air. None of these devices remove allergens. They modify the air you breathe and in some cases, unfortunately very few cases, they help allergy symptoms. You have nothing to lose by trying one of these devices, but don't expect too much from them.

Facts About Exposure To Home Insulation

Some people believe that home insulating material which is made from urea-formaldehyde can produce harmful vapors that trigger allergic symptoms. Until recently, though, no one had surveyed the population to learn the prevalence of this kind of problem.

Out of curiosity, several doctors in Canada studied a group of patients who swore vehemently that urea-formaldehyde vapors from home insulation triggered their asthma. To look into this, the doctors placed their volunteer subjects in a special room and examined them before and after exposing them to urea-formaldehyde vapor. In this way they could do a controlled test for adverse effects.

The surprising result was that only one of the subjects got worse. The rest did not develop asthma despite their previous assertions that urea-formaldehyde had bothered them. The experiment showed that urea-formaldehyde insulation is not as big a problem as was originally believed.

The research also illustrated the fact that a doctor must always double-check his patient's suspicions when it comes to determining what substances are responsible for allergic reactions. If the suspicion is correct, this leads to correct treatment. If the suspicion is wrong, the patient must accept this and with the help of his doctor look elsewhere for the real culprit.

Helpful hint 1: Home insulating material is not the culprit it was thought to be.

Helpful hint 2: No matter how strongly you or your doctor suspect that a particular allergen is responsible for your allergic symptoms, double check your facts.

Helpful hint 3: Assumptions don't count in medicine. They can lead to a false sense of security that you have the correct diagnosis and are following the correct treatment.

Excess Fear of Dust Mites

Dr. Masahiro Sakaguchi from Tokyo's National Institute of Health studied the problem of dust mites in Japan. The study showed that certain people may be overly concerned about dust-mite allergy.

Dust mite particles need especially strong air currents to get into the air. Vacuuming and making the bed create strong air currents that are forceful enough to do this. On the other hand, animal allergens like dog and cat dander enter the air more easily. Everyday foot-traffic in the house will do it.

Dr. Sakaguchi found that during the course of a typical day the level of *animal* allergen in certain homes was up to *eighty times* higher than the level of mite allergen. This is important because allergens that aren't in the air won't reach your respiratory tract and won't bother you.

Helpful hint 1: A longstanding principle of allergy is that you become symptomatic only when allergens enter your respiratory tract. As long as allergens are kept away from you, they cannot affect you.

Helpful hint 2: Dr. Masahiro Sakaguchi's study shows that animal allergens enter the air and gain access to you more easily than dust-mite allergens.

Helpful hint 3: While vacuuming or making beds you stir up the air a lot more and have more to fear from dust mites than pets. When you are at rest and the air is quiet, the opposite is true. You have more to fear from pets than mites.

Helpful hint 4: Although dust mites are important allergens, keep the overall picture in mind and consider the other factors that are important in provoking symptoms besides the mere presence of mites.

Vacuum Vacuum Vacuum

If you are like most people, you think that vacuuming your home is one of the most important ways to allergy-proof your home. Nevertheless and despite what you think, measures that *prevent* exposure and *seal off* allergens *before* they can enter the air are more useful than going through the house each day to get rid of what you could have prevented in the first place.

Still, vacuuming fills a need to do something. So companies have invented various vacuum cleaners to accomodate us.

Vacuum cleaners come in all shapes and sizes. The high-tech type have HEPA filters, charcoal prefilters, and a variety of seals and gadgets to suck up dirt and keep the dirt and dust in the vacuum cannister without spraying it around the room from leaks in the system. One company makes a cleaner with a water trap.

Dr. Ann Woodcock from England studied vacuum cleaners and found that a double-bag collector in an *ordinary* vacuum was as effective as the high-tech devices. Rooms were cleaned and the double bag prevented stirring up particles to the point where the air was a menace to the vacuumer and the patient alike.

Helpful hint 1: Sometimes cheap, simple solutions to a problem are as good as complicated, costly solutions.

Helpful hint 2: It is amazing what a simple, careful study can tell you. You just need someone like Dr. Ann Woodcock who is inquisitive and wasn't willing to accept other peoples' assertions that high-tech equipment is the only way to get rid of dust and dust mites. Thank you, Dr. Woodcock.

5

Allergy To Pets

Allergists have a reputation for disliking pets because we often tell our patients to get rid of their pets. On the other hand, our patients sometimes have what seems to be an unreasonable attachment to pets that are making them as sick as a dog.

Neither allergists nor patients are pig-headed, though.

Both know the best treatment for allergy is avoidance. And both know psychological studies show the companionship of a pet can be beneficial. So if you are allergic to pets, you and your health care professional must balance the good against the bad.

The first of the following studies explains how pets cause allergy. The second one shows that pet-sensitive people can have symptoms in their homes even when they don't own a pet. The third study shows how to wash your pet so your pet doesn't produce allergenic material. And the fourth study shows how to build immunity to your pets so they can't affect you even if you are exposed to them. The fifth shows how tricky it is to treat allergy to pets, and the sixth shows how allergy to cats may not be allergy to cats.

Cat Hair Does Not Cause Allergy

Most of you have heard that cat hair causes allergy. This is not true.

Several doctors at the National Institutes of Health in Bethesda, Maryland, and a group of doctors who work in Germany proved it is not hair but a protein that is found in dander, saliva, and urine that causes allergy symptoms.

To do this bit of research, the doctors collected cat hair. Then they removed the dander and dirt that was stuck to it and rinsed off the saliva where the cats had licked themselves. Lastly, they exposed several volunteer patients to dander, saliva, and *cleaned* cat hair.

The result? The volunteers reacted to dander and saliva. None of them reacted to the hair itself.

By the way, dogs and pet rodents like guinea pigs, hamsters, and mice are also allergenic because of an allergenic protein in their dander, saliva, and urine.

Helpful hint 1: If you are allergic to pets, you are allergic to a protein found in dander, saliva, and urine.

Helpful hint 2: Short-hair cats can produce as much dander as long-hair varieties. Therefore, they can cause just as much allergy.

No One Is Safe From Dogs And Cats

Doctors used to think that if a patient wasn't exposed to a pet, pets couldn't be causing symptoms.

Doctor B. Schwartz in Denmark proved this idea is wrong. She tested homes without pets and found that one-third of them had measurable amounts of animal dander even though there was no pet in the home. Furthermore, the dander was present in quantities that were sufficient to provoke symptoms in highly allergic patients.

Although Dr. Schwartz didn't know how animal dander got into these homes, she speculated that the dander was brought in by clinging to clothing when homeowners visited friends who had pets. The same problem had been found in schools. Children who had pets brought measurable amounts of animal dander with them to school. During the course of the school day the allergen came off their clothes and clung to classroom walls.

Helpful hint 1: These studies show that avoidance of pets is often easier said than done.

Washing Cats Removes Allergenic Dander

Dr. James Wedner of St. Louis, Missouri, performed a great service to cat lovers everywhere. He did an experiment where he washed cats once a month in warm distilled water. He was able to reduce the amount of allergen up to fifty percent after four washings. After nine washings, he was able to reduce the allergen content by seventy-five percent.

I know washing cats isn't easy, but if you are dedicated to your cat and want to do some good for your health, washing your cat is a proven method.

Helpful hint 1: When it comes to animal allergy, avoidance is still the best policy.

Helpful hint 2: No one has studied the effectiveness of washing birds and dogs, so you would have to try it and see if it helps.

Helpful hint 3: If you stop washing your pet, allergens return. So you must keep washing.

Helpful hint 4: If you are allergic to your pet and insist on keeping your pet, shower with a friend.

Allergy Immunizing Injections For Cats And Dogs

For years many allergists offered no solution to pet allergy except avoidance. While avoidance is guaranteed, there are other considerations. Most people love their pets. Additionally, even after giving up a pet, you will still be exposed to neighbors', friends', and relatives' pets.

Now, more and more doctors are willing to give you an option instead of an ultimatum. You may take a series of immunizing injections. Although the injections are time-consuming, they are effective as long as you reach a high dose. This can immunize you enough so that you can keep your pet and not suffer with symptoms.

One reason doctors used to be hesitant to recommend immunizing injections for pets was that they did not have access to the allergy literature and doubted that such injections would work. However, research has confirmed the usefulness of such injections. At a recent allergy meeting Dr. Thomas Van Metre presented a study in which *all* twenty-two patients he treated had significant relief with immunizing injections.

Each week Dr. Van Metre injected an increasing dose of animal dander extract until he reached a maintenance level. At that point he continued injecting his patients once a month. This resulted in enough immunity so that his patients' pets did not trigger allergy symptoms.

But remember, the best treatment is still avoidance. Injections are only an alternative.

Helpful hint 1: If you are allergic to pets, the best treatment is avoidance.

Helpful hint 2: If you insist on having a pet, you can take allergy injections to build your immunity.

Helpful hint 3: If you choose to take allergy injections for pets, your dose of serum must be high enough to achieve a therapeutic effect. Otherwise, you are wasting your time.

Spraying and Tranquilizing Your Cats

Allerpet is a spray that is applied directly onto the cat. Acepromazine is a mild tranquilizer that you give to your cat, *not to yourself*, even though you may sometimes feel like you need a tranquil moment away from the trials and tribulations of constant allergy symptoms. The two products are supposed to neutralize cat allergen. If they worked as advertised, you could keep your cat and be symptom-free.

Dr. Dennis Ownby led a group of researchers who tested both products. He found that neither product reduced the level of cat allergen. You would think this would be the final answer and the end of these products. It isn't. Certain individuals swear these products work for them.

The products are not dangerous, and you may try them if you wish. Just give yourself a set period of time for the trial, a few weeks should be enough. If your allergy symptoms do not stop by the end of the trial, ask your doctor for help. Do not, I repeat *do not* keep using these products in the hope that some day in the future you will wake up cured of cat allergy when your body is telling you that you are not getting better just from spraying and tranquilizing your cat.

Helpful hint 1: If you use Allerpet or Acepromazine, I hope this works for you. But don't depend upon it.

Don't Be Too Quick to Throw Out Your Cat

Dr. Richard Lockey in Florida found patients whose allergies were triggered by extract of cat fleas which are affectionately named Ctenocephalides Felis. (I can't pronounce this either.)

In any case, no matter what you call them, they can evidently cause symptoms and it is certainly worth getting rid of your cat's fleas to see if this helps your allergies.

Helpful hint 1: If you react to cats, you may be reacting to cat allergen, fleas, or both.

Helpful hint 2: Do not use this study as an excuse to keep your cat because you read that fleas and not cats cause allergy symptoms. If your body, your allergy skin tests, and your allergist are telling you that your *cat* is making you sick, listen to what you are being told.

Helpful hint 3: In certain cases, the obvious allergen is not the allergen that bothers you. Other situations where this occurs, for example, are when latex particles attach to powder in surgical gloves and make you think you are allergic to the powder when you are actually allergic to latex, when milk products contaminate supposedly non-milk containing food products and make you mistakenly think you can't be allergic to milk when there are actually hidden milk-contaminants in the "non-milk" containing product, or when mold spores are in the atmosphere at the same time as ragweed pollen and make you think ragweed is the problem when the allergen is really mold.

6

Mold Allergy and How To Avoid Mold

Mold is the mildew or fungus that grows in damp places like bathrooms, near refrigerators, and around air-conditioning units. Some varieties of mold grow where it is relatively dry. So there isn't a universal rule about where you find mold.

Strictly speaking, you are not allergic to mold. You are allergic to the *spores* that molds produce. These are microscopic bits and pieces of mold that are released into the air in the same way grasses, trees, and weeds produce pollen grains which are the components of grasses, trees, and weeds that make you ill.

The first study in this section shows that mold is not where you think it is. The second study explains an inexpensive and environmentally-safe method to get rid of mold. And the third study reports where mold may be hiding in your home.

Mold Is In The Kitchen

Dr. Hector Busaniche from Santa Fe, Argentina, measured the mold levels in various rooms in eight homes. Fifty percent of the mold was in the kitchens due to moisture around refrigerators and sinks. Thirty percent was found in bedrooms, and twenty percent was in bathrooms. These findings were a surprise. Like most people, he had expected bathrooms to be the major source of mold.

When I ask my patients to remove mold, most of them deny they even have mold in their homes. They don't realize you cannot see mold with the naked eye unless there are thousands of colonies clumped together. Of those people who admit to mold in the home, they, like Dr. Busaniche, think of the bathroom first. This study shows that mold is everywhere.

Helpful hint 1: Mold is found throughout the home. But, the most common location for mold is in the kitchen.

Heat Kills Mold

Dr. Jeff Miller, who practices allergy in Connecticut, studied a method of killing mold with heat. Although some molds can be heat resistant, heat killed ninety-nine percent of the molds Dr. Miller tested. He accomplished this by running a portable space heater, closing the door to the room, and heating for about forty-eight hours. Of course, you've got to repeat this from time to time to prevent mold from regrowing, but heat is environmentally safe so there is no danger from using this technique.

You can also use chemicals, called fungicides, to kill mold. These chemicals may be applied to ceilings, walls, floors, and even rugs. They can last for months at a time, depending on the type of chemical you use.

Helpful hint 1: If you use heat to kill molds, you must re-heat on a regular basis.

Helpful hint 2: You can purchase fungicides from companies that sell allergy products or from local stores and plant-nurseries.

Mold Under the Rug

Dr. Thomas Platts-Mills and others have discovered that mold grows under rugs that are laid over cement slabs. This is insidious. You cannot see the mold, yet the spores are discharged into the air just as easily as if the molds were in plain sight.

Furthermore, vacuuming stirs up the mold particles. This can trigger ugly allergy attacks, including difficult-to-treat asthma. Just walking over a rug can create air currents that bring mold to the top.

So if you are allergic to mold, you must deal with it harshly. Don't hold back. Get rid of it.

Helpful hint 1: If you are allergic to mold and your rugs are laid on a concrete slab, you should pull up the rug or treat the rug regularly with a fungicide.

7

Food Allergy

Food sensitivity usually causes skin and gastrointestinal symptoms. However, foods can also cause respiratory symptoms, headaches, fatigue, and even death.

Some physicians won't think about foods as possibly responsible for certain symptoms because medical schools don't teach too much about food reactions. This is unfortunate because if a health care professional isn't aware that foods can cause various symptoms, he won't think of investigating. The result would be a missed opportunity to find out what's wrong.

On the other hand patients err, too, either because they are too hasty to conclude that foods are responsible for certain health problems or too stubborn to look into the possibility when their doctor suggests that foods might be a contributing factor.

The first two studies show you cannot assume you are allergic to foods. You must do careful tests to be sure. The third study shows how dangerous food allergy can be. The fourth study describes a drug that can alleviate certain types of food allergy. The next study shows that food allergy can cause arthritis, which was an amazing finding when it was first described. The next study explains how foods can cause migraine headaches. Then there is a word about avoidance of foods, what kinds of non-allergenic infant formulas have been developed, and how you can react to a food even if you don't eat the food. Next are a warning about severe allergic shock, called anaphylaxis, and how you need to be prepared for emergencies, a disturbing problem that occurred due to a biologically-engineered food, and finally several reports about life-threatening food reactions, which are the kinds of reactions that give allergists indigestion.

Sugar Allergy Findings

Dr. Kathy Mahan studied sixteen children who had been diagnosed by their doctors as allergic to sugar. She hoped to learn what kinds of symptoms they had and how she could help such patients.

When Dr. Mahan fed the sixteen children sugar-containing foods such as candy, nine of the sixteen did not become aggressive, overly active, loud, or argumentative, which were the symptoms that had brought the children to their doctors' attention and which everyone was blaming on sugar allergy. The remaining seven had a fifteen percent increase in their activity level when they ate sugar, but fifteen percent can't be considered too much of a difference when it comes to comparing behavior in active, growing children.

Nevertheless, being a good scientist Dr. Mahan wanted to double-check her findings on the seven who reacted. She wanted to make sure they weren't cheating. To do this, she conducted another experiment where she put sugar in capsules to disguise the taste. Then she fed the capsules to the seven children whose behavior had changed. Much to her dismay, when the children could not tell they were getting sugar, they didn't react. This showed that the seven children had reacted only when they knew they were expected to react.

Thus, Dr. Mahan's experiment was a failure. She could not find children who were truly allergic to sugar.

In conclusion, Dr. Mahan observed that half of the children she had studied did not react *even when they knew* they were eating sugar. The other half reacted *only if they knew* they were eating sugar.

Helpful hint 1: It may be tempting to blame bad behavior on allergy to sugar. However, studies show that blaming bad behavior on sugar allergy is probably just an excuse to avoid looking for the true cause.

Helpful hint 2: There may be rare individuals who react badly to sugar, but Dr. Kathy Mahan has shown that sugar allergy is very much over-diagnosed. Her experiment should make us ask why some of us are so eager to blame difficult behavior problems on a food such as sugar instead of trying to figure out the true reason.

Good News For Kids With Food Allergies

For the past fifteen years Dr. Allan Bock has studied food allergy in children. His research is full of good news.

For three years he kept track of 500 children who were three years of age or under. He found that forty percent of them (about 200 children) were reported by their parents and doctors to have had food reactions.

Of these 200 children, sixty-five (thirty-three percent) proved allergic to fruits. Their reactions were brief and usually lasted only a few hours. Twenty-six children (twelve percent) reacted to milk, soybean, peanut, egg, wheat or chocolate. The remaining one-hundred and nine children (fifty-five perecent) didn't react to anything. The diagram on the next page illustrates this.

200 Children *Reported* Allergic

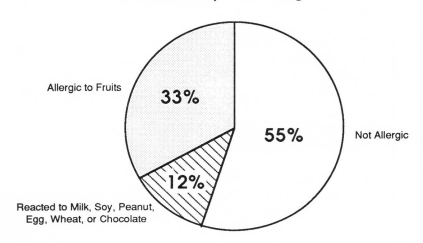

One year later Dr. Bock reviewed what had happened to the children who had reacted. He found they were no longer allergic. The offending food had been re-introduced into their diet without ill effect.

Helpful hint 1: Of all the children under three who are believed by their parents and doctors to have food allergies, thirty-three percent are allergic to fruits. However, their sensitivity does not usually last more than a few months. Another twelve percent of children are allergic to milk, soy, peanut, egg, wheat, or chocolate. And fifty-five percent of supposedly allergic children are not allergic to anything. Thus fifty-five percent of food-allergic children have been misdiagnosed.

Helpful hint 2: A lot of parents and doctors are incorrectly blaming foods for causing various symptoms in children when something else is at fault.

Helpful hint 3: Even when foods cause allergy symptoms, the foods can almost always be re-introduced into a child's diet after a few months without causing adverse problems.

Helpful hint 4: Most children who are thought to have food allergy do not have food allergy.

Not Eating The Food You Are Allergic To Can Kill You

Avoidance is the number one, favorite treatment of allergists. This always works. Guaranteed.

When it comes to food avoidance, this would seem to be simple. Don't eat the food and nothing can happen.

However, Dr. S. Figueroa working with Dr. Dennis Ownby in Michigan discovered that steam coming from cooking foods can contain enough allergen to cause a reaction.

Dr. Figueroa boiled two shrimp, collected the steam, and found shrimp allergen in the steam. Although the amount of allergen was small, about fifty times less than in the water used to boil the shrimp, a highly sensitive person could react. So food-sensitive people need to be especially careful.

Although the study on boiled shrimp is recent, allergists have known about the problem of trace contaminants for quite some time from bitter experience with peanut allergy. Companies often make batches of peanut- and non-peanut-containing products in the same large industrial container. In between production runs, they wash, rinse, and clean, but they don't always do a thorough job. Traces of peanut protein can be left behind between one batch and another, and this can cause allergic reactions in unsuspecting people.

Helpful hint 1: All that nonsense about a word to the wise being sufficient is nonsense. A word is not enough. If you are highly sensitive to a particular food, you need to be constantly on guard and learn as much as you can about the foods you eat. You may even have to write to the manufacturer and carry emergency medication with you in case you have an inadvertent reaction.

New Drug To Treat Food Allergy

Many years ago a British pharmaceutical company developed an anti-allergy drug called cromolyn that strengthens Mast cells so they do not release their histamine even though they are coated with too much IgE antibody. You could think of cromolyn as a plastic bag that holds histamine inside the cells. It isn't really plastic, but the effect would be the same.

Now the company has put this drug in capsules for intestinal use. The name of the drug is Gastrocrom, and before you get your hopes too high, I must tell you it doesn't work for everyone. However it is worth trying because it is not absorbed into the body and is perfectly safe.

Before trying Gastrocrom, make sure you have food allergy. There are many conditions that mimic food allergy such as lactose intolerance which is due to lack of the enzyme, *lactase*, that digests milk sugar which is *lactose*.

Another intolerance is associated with tyramine in cheese. This intolerance causes headaches. This is a metabolic intolerance and not an allergic reaction.

There are many myths and misunderstandings in the field of food allergy. For your own health and safety you should consult a physician who is knowledgeable about food allergy and is willing to work with you. Don't succumb to easy-sounding blood and skin tests that are being promoted these days. They are unreliable and can lead you to useless or, more importantly, dangerous treatments.

Finally, remember that the best treatment for food allergy is avoidance. However, you are welcome to try Gastrocrom. Just do it under your doctor's supervision. If used prior to eating, this may *prevent* food reactions.

Helpful hint 1: The key to treating food reactions is obtaining the correct diagnosis of the *type* of reaction you have. For example, treatment of food-intolerance as if it was food-allergy is doomed to failure and visa versa.

Helpful hint 2: If food allergy is responsible for your symptoms, you *might* obtain relief by taking a new drug called Gastrocrom.

Helpful hint 3: Many food reactions are blamed on allergy when in fact the reactions are due to other mechanisms.

Milk Allergy Shown To Cause Arthritis

Dr. Richard Panush at the University of Florida discovered an amazing food reaction. He found an elderly woman who suffered from arthritis due to ingestion of milk.

Over the years there have been numerous claims in health books, magazines, newspaper articles, and even from certain health care professionals about food allergy causing arthritis. However, the majority of experiments that allegedly prove that foods cause arthritis are so uncontrolled and poorly done that no scientist in good conscience could believe the claims.

I've read Dr. Panush's study, and it is believable!

The patient in question suffered with typical arthritis symptoms such as joint stiffness and swelling. When she ceased ingesting milk products, her symptoms stopped. To make certain this wasn't a case of mistaken identity, Dr. Panush double-checked her in a hospital under supervised conditions where he disguised several foods so his patient did not know what she was eating and therefore could not be biased.

This technique is called a blinded-controlled study, and Dr. Panush showed that his patient's observations about milk were correct. However, she thought two other foods aggravated her arthritis, too. A blinded test for the other two foods showed that she was wrong about the other two foods.

Discovering a patient whose arthritis was due to milk was an unexpected and fascinating observation. But this doesn't mean *your* arthritis is due to milk allergy. In any situation where you or your doctors suspect a food is responsible for a particular symptom, you must work *together* with your doctor to prove beyond doubt that food is the causative factor.

Dr. Panush practices in the arthritis clinic of a large teaching hospital in Florida where he sees many cases of arthritis each year. After he discovered that a food caused this patient's arthritis, he looked extra carefully for similar cases. Unfortunately, he and his colleagues have not found a similar case after three years of searching.

Helpful hint 1: Your doctors have to be open minded and listen to you when you tell them what you think is making you ill. Then they have to help you figure out if your observations are correct.

Helpful hint 2: Of the hundreds of thousands of cases of arthritis in the United States, very few are due to milk allergy. So do not stop arthritis or any other treatment on the slim chance that food allergy is the sole cause of your arthritis. Instead, consult your doctor, be willing to look into the possibility, and abide by the facts.

Migraine Headaches Due To Food Allergy Leads Doctors To An Entirely New Disease -- Pseudo Food Allergy

Migraine headaches are a pain in the neck (as well as other parts of the head) because they are difficult to treat. Many times doctors look high and low to find a cause and come up empty handed. So when a doctor discovers a new place to look, we all get interested.

Dr. Philip Fireman, from Pittsburgh, Pennsylvania, found a patient who developed migraine headaches soon after eating peanut, soy, corn, and beef. Several sophisticated x-ray tests (tomography and ultrasonography) confirmed his diagnosis.

Although Dr. Fireman was excited because he thought he would now be able to help the tens of thousands of migraine sufferers by finding hidden food allergy, he had a difficult time finding other migraine patients whose migraine was due to foods. So he probably became discouraged. I wouldn't blame him. I'd be discouraged, too.

In fact, the problem of blaming symptoms such as migraine headaches, fatigue, overweight, difficulty thinking, and hyperactivity, to name just a few conditions that certain health care professionals blame on food allergy when food allergy isn't at fault, has created an entirely new disease called *Pseudo* Food Allergy.

This new condition was reported by Dr. Gordon Sussman at the University of Toronto. Mistaken diagnosis of food allergy is a widespread problem because many people want to believe there is an easy answer to a complicated medical problem. Unwilling to do the hard work necessary to diagnose food allergy through elimination diets, these people rely on skin and blood tests even though repeated studies have shown that skin and blood tests for food allergy are highly inaccurate and misleading.

Typically, the patient is talked into paying for "modern" blood tests, given a computer printout of foods that showed up on the test, and told to avoid the foods that are on the list. No attempt is made to double-check the test results with an elimination or provocative-challenge diet. Instead, the person is sent home to struggle with a diet that is usually of no benefit. In fact many people become depressed. Here they are following a diet as well as they can, their symptoms are still there, and they begin to fault themselves. The real fault is the vain hope that skin and blood tests for foods are accurate. If a person doesn't have low self-esteem from being ill and unable to function before he heard of food allergy tests, he will certainly develop low self-esteem when he keeps blaming himself for lack of success with his "scientifically-proven" diet.

Helpful hint 1: There are many interesting individual case reports of people who suffer all kinds of symptoms due to food allergy. However, most of these cases are isolated. So, think twice before blaming food allergy for *your* symptoms just because you heard someone with similar symptoms had food allergy or because a skin or high-tech blood test says you have food allergy.

Helpful hint 2: On the other hand, you may be the one person in ten or twenty who feels better avoiding a particular food. So if your doctor suggests doing a food diet (as opposed to skin or blood tests) to look into possible food allergy, be willing to try.

A Word About Avoidance Of Foods

When it comes to food allergy, avoidance is the best policy. However, you usually need to be an ace-detective to avoid foods rigorously. No matter how diligent you are, you can still make a mistake.

Dr. John Yunginger from Rochester, Minnesota, studied a case where a milk-allergic person ate a sorbet desert that was labeled kosher *and* milk free. Relying on the label, the sorbet seemed safe. However, just minutes after ingestion Dr. Yunginger's patient experienced hives and difficulty breathing. Upon chemical analysis of the sorbet, Dr. Yunginger found it contained milk protein contaminants.

Most of you are aware that labels and advertising cannot always be trusted. For food allergic individuals, trusting labels can mean the difference between life and death.

Helpful hint 1: If you are allergic to foods, don't trust labels.

Non-Allergenic Formula for Infants

Cows' milk allergy affects one percent of infants. In the earliest attempts companies made alternative formulas from plants which created a soybean-based formula and animal byproducts which created a meat-based formula. Next the manufacturers learned how to heat cows' milk with enzymes to make them less allergenic. The popular brands of heat-and-enzyme-treated milk come from casein (Nutramigen, Pregestimil, and Alimentum) or whey (Good Start, Ultrafiltered Good Start, and Alfare). All of these are available throughout the United States.

Dr. Robert Schwartz at the University of Rochester Medical Center studied twenty-three children who were milk-allergic. He was never at a loss to find a formula for a child. But he couldn't find a formula that was foolproof. Certain infants tolerated one kind, and others had to be given another kind. The outcome of this research led the American Academy of Pediatrics to establish the following guidelines. *Non-allergenic* was to be reserved for a formula that *all* infants could tolerate. *Hypo-allergenic* meant that *ninety percent* of infants could tolerate the product. As Dr. Schwartz showed, all of the currently-available formulas for infants are to be considered *hypo*-allergenic.

Helpful hint 1: At the present time we do not have a *non*-allergenic infant formula, only *hypo*-allergenic.

Helpful hint 2: If your infant is allergic to milk, you will probably have to try several hypo-allergenic formulas in order to find the one your child can tolerate.

Helpful hint 3: Even modern science has limits on what it can accomplish.

Cross-Reacting Foods

Cross-reacting foods sounds like foods that are angry at each other. In fact, it is the opposite. Cross-reacting means the foods behave the same way.

Dr. Consuela Fernandez studied several patients who had shock-like reactions to herbal tea, camomile-based ointments, and sunflower seeds. Each of these substances belongs to the Compositae family of plants. Ragweed, the major allergy provoking weed of the fall pollen season in the United States, is in this family, too.

Thus, although the above foodstuffs appear to be different, herbal tea, sunflower seeds, and so forth, they clearly share an identical allergic constituent. Other examples of cross-reactivity occur when people who are allergic to latex react to bananas, those allergic to frogs' legs react to codfish, or those sensitive to peanuts react to stringbeans.

To make matters more complicated, Dr. R. van Whee from Amsterdam studied several patients who had house-dust mite allergy and suddenly developed asthma after eating snails. His interest was piqued because he apparently likes snails and this cross-reaction had not been reported before. Using complex molecular analysis, he investigated and discovered that house dust mites cross react with snails. He then theorized that exposure to house dust mites had caused his subjects to become sensitive to snails. Dr. van Whee further warned that giving injections to immunize a person for house dust mite (which is a treatment you will read about in a later chapter) may sensitize you to snails.

Helpful hint 1: By learning what family of allergens you are allergic to, your doctors can often predict that you will be sensitive to other, seemingly different, substances.

Helpful hint 2: Genetic research has given us the tools to find the specific molecules that cause allergic reactions. Eventually this will allow us to identify the common denominator in certain foods that cause reactions even though the foods may look, feel, and taste differently. For example, tropomyosin has been identified as one of the molecules that cause shrimp allergy. Cysteine protease is one of the molecules that cause dust mite allergy.

Helpful hint 3: Until cross-reactivity is completely sorted out and defined, eater beware!

Watch Out For Biologically-Engineered Foods

Many scientists are hard at work studying how to make the foods we eat faster growing, drought tolerant, resistant to disease, and more nutritious. They hope this research will pay off in lower cost, improved quality, and increased yield. As you can probably guess, the key to success will be applying genetic engineering principles to plants in the same way doctors apply genetic engineering to help overcome human disease.

Despite the obvious advantages of improved food quality and more abundant supplies, some people fear that gene engineering may create a nightmare like the Hollywood horror movies where tomatoes go on a rampage and kill human beings. While the killer-tomato theory is far-fetched and unrealistic, although the 1950's movie about this wasn't so bad, fear of allergic problems due to bio-engineered foods is a reality.

Brazil nuts are high in methionine which is a chemical that contains sulfur. Soybeans, on the other hand, are low in methionine. So certain scientists decided to put the part of the Brazil nut gene that makes methionine into soybean seeds. This would produce a soybean high in sulfur and make soybeans more nutritious.

J.A. Nordlee led the experimental team that did this. However, to allergists' dismay the transferred Brazil nut gene that produced the extra sulfur also contained the allergically-reactive Brazil nut gene.

The bottom line is that if a person is allergic to Brazil nuts and eats the new and wonderful soybeans, he might suffer a fatal allergic reaction. You could say that this is the killer-tomato story come true.

Helpful hint 1: Bioengineered foods can have advantages as well as disadvantages.

Helpful hint 2: A solution to an agricultural problem such as how to grow a disease-resistant or a more nutritious food may cause unintended consequences.

Helpful hint 3: It may not be wise to mess with Mother Nature.

Infants Threaten To Overturn Standard Allergy Theory

Allergy theory states that higher than normal levels of IgE antibody cause allergic reactions. In order to make high levels of IgE antibody the person must be exposed to various allergens. The process of exposure to allergen and making too much IgE antibody is called *sensitization*. Thus, you can see how it would be impossible for a person to be sensitized if he wasn't exposed to an allergen. And in fact it usually requires *multiple* exposures over a period of years to develop allergy.

Suddenly along came some infants who were born in Italy and had been exclusively breast-fed and seemed to react to cows' milk on what seemed to be their first eating of cows' milk. These infants, who couldn't even talk, were threatening to overturn standard allergy theory.

Well, I can tell you that allergists were dismayed by these infants. If what had happened to them was true, it meant allergists had to develop a new theory.

Dr. Arnaldo Cantani, who is a professor in Italy, came to the rescue. He studied these infants backwards and forwards and discovered that they had been fed cows' milk formula in the nursery on certain nights before the mothers had left the hospital. Allergists everywhere breathed a sigh of relief.

There is another situation where your infant may ingest allergens and you won't know about it. Dr. Martha DeBolt asked nursing mothers to eat peanuts and tested their breast milk for the presence of peanut protein. She detected peanut protein from three to five hours later. This shows that what a mother eats when she is breast-feeding can pass to her child, sensitize the infant, and lead to allergy on what might mistakenly appear to be the first exposure.

Helpful hint 1: Allergy theory is still correct. You cannot react *allergically* if this is *truly* your first exposure.

Helpful hint 2: Your first exposures to allergens create a state of sensitivity. In this process you build your IgE to higher than normal levels. *Subsequent* exposures cause symptoms.

Helpful hint 3: Breast feeding does not necessarily protect an infant from developing food allergy. The nursing mother needs to be careful what she eats, too.

Chicken Soup Causes Near-Fatal Reaction

At many of the scientific meetings doctors report cases of sudden death as a result of severe reactions to one food or another. I'm sorry to tell you this, but with each passing year there are more and more reports. So the problem is getting worse, not better. In fact there are so many cases that it can take a half-day seminar to discuss them. The official term for these kinds of reactions is sudden or fatal anaphylaxis.

At one recent meeting Dr. Robert Schwartz presented an interesting case that illustrates the problem. A seven year old child was recovering from pneumonia and was fed chicken soup. The child stopped breathing. Fortunately this occurred in the hospital where the child was quickly revived. Upon investigation the doctors discovered that the chicken soup contained traces of milk. The child had been known to be allergic to milk, but no one suspected chicken soup would contain milk.

Helpful hint 1: There are many jokes about the curative properties of chicken soup. In some cases, though, chicken soup can be hazardous to your health.

Helpful hint 2: If you have food allergy, being in the hospital can be hazardous to your health because the dietary department may not be as astute as you or your family in reading labels and figuring out what is safe to eat.

Watch Your Pizza Topping

Dr. Samuel Lehrer from New Orleans investigated patients who reacted to pizza. What puzzled him was that the patients knew they were allergic to fish, had been educated on how to avoid fish, and had been compliant. This was not a group of rebellious teenagers trying to prove they could eat fish and get away with it. They were responsible adults who were careful about what they ate.

Dr. Lehrer found that these patients had ordered a pizza with pepperoni meat topping. They felt this was safe. They didn't realize that some restaurants use a substitute meat called surimi that tastes like meat but is made from fish. The topping that caused the problem in Dr. Lehrer's patients was an imitation sausage made from pollock. Other meat substitutes are made from haddock, hake and cod.

This is just another example of how scary life is for food-sensitive patients. They can never be complacent about what they are eating.

Helpful hint 1: These days many companies manufacture imitation substitute-foods that are made from a variety of ingredients. You may have no clue about the contents. You need to be prepared for an allergic reaction and have a plan of action. Discuss this with your doctor.

Helpful hint 2: Be prepared in case you are allergic to foods. Carry emergency epinephrine (adrenalin) and an antihistamine whereever you go. You don't want to be a statistic at a scientific meeting of allergists

8

Food-Additive Allergy

While allergy to foods has existed since man first appeared on earth, allergy to food-additives is a modern problem. We created additives so we could transport foods, keep them fresh, and make them appeal to our sense of taste, sight, and smell.

For susceptible individuals food-additive reactions are a nightmare. There are dozens of different preservatives, additives, flavorings, and chemicals. Between manufacturing needs, government regulations, cancer scares, public changes in taste, and what is current in nutrition, the various food companies frequently change the ingredients they use to make their products, often without advance warning.

The following studies illustrate true and false reports about food additives. The first describes what we know about a certain kind of food-additive allergy. The second case shows how a story can be distorted and blown out of proportion.

Treatment For Food Additive Allergy

Restaurant salads can provoke asthma. The salad literally takes your breath away. Individuals with this susceptibility may also break out in hives from head to foot. These reactions are dramatic, severe, and can be difficult to stop. In several cases fatalities have occurred.

The cause of these reactions has been traced to a preservative called bisulfite. One out of ten asthmatic adults is said to be sulfite-sensitive. Allergists have known about this for many years, but they hadn't found a solution other than to recommend avoidance.

Now, Dr. Donald Stevenson at Scripps Clinic in La Jolla, California, has found a way to treat such individuals. He administered the very medication that caused the reaction in the first place, but he did this according to a special schedule. He is fine-tuning the method and the rest of us in clinical practice hope he finishes soon. But until then, the best policy is avoidance.

Certain people develop a similar sensitivity to aspirin, yellow food dyes called tartrazine, pain killers, and several anti-inflammatory drugs such as Naprosyn, Motrin, and Ibuprofen. So anyone who is sensitive to bisulfite should talk to their doctor. They may have to avoid other chemicals and drugs, too.

On the other hand, this problem can be overdramatized. Newspaper and TV reporters often blow the issue out of proportion. Some writers want to make you think *everyone* reacts to these chemicals. In fact, only a few individuals are affected. For those of you who are susceptible, of course, this is a serious problem. For the rest of you, though, you needn't be concerned. Furthermore, there is no evidence that regular ingestion of these chemicals makes you become allergic to them unless you are one of the one in ten who was going to become allergic anyway.

Additional Help Is On The Way

In 1986 the United States Food and Drug Administration acknowledged the problem of sulfite sensitivity and banned the use of these types of chemicals on fresh fruit and vegetables. The FDA also required that sulfite-containing packages be labelled. Nevertheless, don't depend on voluntary compliance by restaurants, food manufacturers, and supermarkets. The consequences of a slip up on their part can endanger your life.

Helpful hint 1: If you have aspirin sensitivity, there is a possibility you can be desensitized.

Helpful hint 2: When someone warns you about a medical problem, ask them what percent of people have the problem. This is one way you can keep fearful news in perspective and not become paranoid over every ominous report that appears in a newspaper, magazine, or television.

Helpful hint 3: If you are sensitive to sulfites, you cannot trust that every restaurant in the United States knows about and complies with the 1986 FDA ban on sulfites.

Dr. Ben Feingold Denies That Food Additives Cause Hyperactivity

Dr. Ben Feingold was one of the first physicians who made a specialty out of practicing allergy. Over the years he made many important contributions to our knowledge. One of his ideas, however, became controversial. This was his theory that food additives and preservatives caused behavioral changes in children.

When you have an idea in science, others try to repeat your studies to see if your idea is true. Scientists don't like inconsistency. They want theories to work or not work. No in-between. For example, when Isaac Newton told the world that the universe is ruled by gravity and that objects are pulled to earth based on the law of gravity, other scientists would have found it hard to accept the law if it did not operate twenty-four hours a day. They would have ridiculed Newton's concept if one day gravity pulled objects toward earth and another day sent the same objects shooting into space.

This is one of the reasons Dr. Feingold's theory became controversial. Other doctors who prescribed his diet discovered that only *certain* children improved.

Another problem that made the Feingold diet controversial was confusion about what kinds of symptoms that food additives caused. I had read and heard that the Feingold diet was to treat *hyper*activity. One day I came across a statement in a respected medical journal where Dr. Feingold was quoted as saying his diet did *not* treat hyperactivity. I couldn't believe this so I wrote him to ask if he had been quoted correctly. To my surprise he told me he had. His letter said that he was often misquoted and that his experience showed that additives and coloring agents caused *hypo*activity, which is the exact opposite of *hyper*activity.

Helpful hint 1: According to Dr. Ben Feingold, food additives can cause *hypo*-activity in *certain* individuals.

Helpful hint 2: Even when you think you understand a person's ideas, you sometimes need to ask a second time to be certain you had it right.

Helpful hint 3: If you think you or your child react to food additives, you may try the Feingold diet. If there is significant improvement, follow the diet. If not, stop the diet.

9

Medication and Treatment for Eye, Nasal, and Sinus Symptoms

Sneezing, stuffy nose, runny nose, postnasal drainage, itch-watery eyes, blocked ears, and headaches are common allergy symptoms. When they occur during a particular season, they are called hayfever. When they occur throughout the year, they are called perennial allergic rhinitis. Eye symptoms are called allergic conjunctivitis. Headaches may be due to allergic sinusitis. So the name changes depending on which particular symptoms you have and what time of year you suffer.

There are a variety of drugs that alleviate these upper respiratory symptoms. Typical medications are antihistamines, decongestants, cortisone-steroids, and a special type of drug called an anti-allergy preparation.

The medications come in various forms: tablets, capsules, liquids, sprays, injections, and inhalants. Unfortunately I am not going to be able to tell you which drug is best for you because I don't know your story, what you are allergic to, what kind of lifestyle you lead, and how your body will respond.

All is not lost, however. Your doctor can help you figure this out. He or she can take a history, examine you, perform, tests, and put the whole story together. This will lead to a treatment plan that should start you on the road to good health.

In the meantime, read the following studies which explain how allergy-drugs work, how to use them, and what kinds of side effects to watch for. You will read about a new hope for sinus headaches, a surprising treatment for itchy-watery eyes, and a method to help you avoid allergens. You will read about the strongest antihistamine known to mankind (sorry, *human*kind still sounds awkward to me), how an antihistamine can make asthma worse, an antihistamine that was advertised as not making people sleepy, an antihistamine that can last all day, how drug companies can make an old drug seem like a new drug, six kinds of adverse drug reactions, and the amazing story about how doctors hope to predict side effects of drugs before they happen.

New Hope For Sinus Headache Sufferers

There are uncountable numbers of people who have headaches due to sinus disease. Dr. Sheldon Spector selected a typical group of such patients and investigated them thoroughly.

Your sinuses are located deep within your skull bone. The only way your doctors can tell what is happening in them is either open your skull, which is ridiculous because this is a major surgical operation, or order an X-ray, which can be costly.

Dr. Spector hoped he could find a simple, inexpensive alternative such as taking a careful history, performing a quick physical examination, looking at your sinuses with a flashlight in a dark room, which is a technique used to visualize fluid in the sinuses, ordering a blood test, or obtaining nasal and sinus bacterial cultures. He even tried special fiberoptic instruments. Lastly, he and his co-workers tried to feel the sinuses by pressing over the forehead and cheeks.

After all this work, Dr. Spector discovered that *none* of these methods reveals what is happening in the sinuses. This forced him to conclude that an X-ray was the only practical way to "see" the state of the sinus cavities since a major operation on your skull is overkill.

Dr. Spector was discouraged. At first this might strike you as discouraging, too. On the contrary, the study is encouraging. It shows that no matter how severe are your headaches, unless a sinus x-ray shows that your sinuses are infected or otherwise malfunctioning, you may not have sinus disease. And if you do not have sinus disease, you can stop being treated for sinus disease. Instead, you can start to look into what is *really* causing your headaches and be treated accordingly. You will accomplish nothing by taking sinus treatments when you don't have sinus disease.

Helpful hint 1: If you do not *truly* have sinus disease, there is no point being treated for sinus disease. Instead, find out what you do have and treat *that*.

Helpful hint 2: By the time you finish this book, I hope you learn that you should not be treated for one disease when your problem is caused by another disease.

Treatment Found For Itchy, Watery Eyes

One of the symptoms of hayfever is itchy, watery eyes. Two doctors from the Netherlands discovered a new way to stop these symptoms. The doctors noticed that seventy-five percent of their patients who had eye symptoms improved even though the doctors ignored the eye problem and just treated the nasal symptoms.

Dr. Zdenek Pelikan, one of the doctors who performed the study, proposed that when the nasal membrane is strongly affected by allergy, the inflammation caused by the allergic reaction can travel from the nose to the eyes through the tear ducts. These are tubes that connect the nose and the eyes. They ordinarily carry tears downward from the eyes, but being open there is no reason inflammation cannot travel backwards in the other direction. So if you are finding it difficult to control allergy in your eyes, you may have better luck if you ignore your eyes and treat your nasal allergies.

Helpful hint 1: Some patients who have allergic conjunctivitis (the official name for eye allergy) are symptomatic due to retrograde nasal allergy.

Helpful hint 2: If you have persistent allergy symptoms despite treatment, consult your doctor so he can figure out why you are not responding.

Newest Way To Avoid Allergens

Do you know what priming is? It is a concept that was promulgated years ago, and I want you to learn about it. It will help you understand a new philosophy about how to avoid allergens.

When you are allergic to two or more substances, exposure to one substance will prime you to be more sensitive to the other. For example, if one morning you walk among trees and return home to your cat, the exposure to two allergens (trees and cat) on the same day will make you more ill than if you were exposed to only one allergen on that particular day. You could say that tree pollen started your ball rolling and cat exposure kept it rolling until there was an allergy avalanche.

Another way to look at priming is to think of the straw that broke the camel's back. When you pile one straw on top of another, the camel will bear the load until the breaking point. When the last straw is placed, the one that is too much, the poor camel's back will break. At first you may think that the *last* straw was the one responsible for breaking the camel's back, but *each* straw played a role.

Priming is a fancy way of saying that it takes a *combination* and *accumulation* of allergens to stretch you beyond your tolerance. The more allergens you are allergic to and the more contact you have with those allergens the worse you will be.

But if you look at the situation from the treatment point of view, you can see that you may be able to obtain satisfactory relief with only a few changes. Just as all the straws contribute equally to breaking a camel's back and just as you can lighten a camel's load by removing *any* of the straws, you can remove a few of the straws (the allergens) that are breaking *your* back and see if this does the job. More improtantly, you can choose which straws you wish to remove. Of course the more straws you remove the lighter your load, but the point is that most patients don't have to remove *every* last wisp in order to feel better.

This is a long-winded way of stating that you may not have to undertake every known form of allergy treatment for each and every allergen to which your are sensitive.

When Dr. John Conell studied priming, he found that certain allergy sufferers who were allergic to multiple allergens felt remarkably better when they merely made a few changes in their lifestyle or even partially limited their exposure to certain allergens. More treatment wasn't worth more effort. For example, Dr. Conell's patients averaged about seventy-five to eighty percent relief. For them, this was more than enough. They felt a lot better and hadn't had to turn their lives inside out to cope with their allergies. Compare this approach to the old way where doctors encouraged you to do everything possible.

The Old Way To Think Of Allergy Treatment

In the old days allergists wrote a prescription that sometimes sought to control your entire life.

- If you're allergic to trees, move to the beach.
- If you're allergic to ragweed, go to Europe.
- If you're allergic to cats, get rid of your cats.
- If you're allergic to grass, stay indoors.
- If you have asthma, quit sports.
- If you're allergic to dust, scrub the house daily.

Although this all-or-none advice is technically correct, it can create its own problems. There are many variables of lifestyle, habits, and personality traits that make knee-jerk answers inappropriate. This is why computers can never replace a good old-fashioned doctor who takes your *overall* best interests into consideration when advising you what to do.

The New Way To Think Of Allergy Treatment

Priming shows you a sensible way to overcome allergy. Previously you might have thought you had no choices. Your allergist would tell you your sensitivities, expect you to avoid the offending allergens, and automatically start a series of allergy injections.

In the new approach, you and your doctor (that is, *both* of you) consider the *entire* picture; your allergens, symptoms, lifestyle, and preferences. Then, between the two of you, you decide which of your various allergens to treat. If you can do a good job on a few of them, you may improve so much that, like Dr. Conell's patients, you can ignore several allergens that are difficult to deal with. You may be surprised how much better you feel after a few minor adjustments.

Helpful hint 1: You can often do a few simple things for a limited number of allergens and feel so much better that undertaking additional treatment is not worth the extra effort.

Helpful hint 2: Don't let people tell you what to do for your allergy. Instead choose which of the various treatment possibilities you wish to undertake. Do them carefully. If this doesn't help you, though, be ready to do more.

Helpful hint 3: The medically and scientifically best treatment may not be the *personally* best treatment for *you*.

Strongest Antihistamine Known to Mankind

The truth is finally out! The strongest antihistamine known to mankind is Doxepin. This isn't even an antihistamine. It's an antidepressant. Pharmacologists have calculated that Doxepin is over 100 time stronger than Benadryl, which is one of the strongest antihistamines we have.

Skeptics might say that if an antidepressant is the strongest antihistamine, this proves allergy is a psychological problem. However, many drugs have a dual purpose. Aspirin relieves fever and arthritis. Sympathomimetic drugs decongest your nose, relieve asthma, and help you lose weight. So dual-purpose isn't unique to Doxepin. The molecule is just shaped in a way that allows it to block histamine receptors in addition to performing its antidepressant effect. The fact that Doxepin has a shape that allows it to block histamine does not mean that allergy is a psychological disease.

Helpful hint 1: The drug with the strongest antihistamine-like property is an antidepressant.

Helpful hint 2: Many drugs have a dual purpose.

Helpful hint 3: Suffering with chronic allergy may make you feel depressed, but the preferred treatment is not taking antidepressants. Instead, avoid allergens, use standard antihistamines for symptomatic relief, or build your immunity with allergy injections.

Antihistamines Can Make Asthma Worse

Antihistamines are known for drying nasal mucus. So some physicians hesitate to recommend them to patients who have asthma for fear that the antihistamines will dry the lung mucus and make the asthma worse. There are warnings about this possibility in nearly every medical textbook.

Upon reviewing the original research, however, allergists discovered that the studies had not been done carefully. So despite the dire textbook-warnings, allergists got in the habit of prescribing antihistamines when their asthmatics complained of nasal allergy. The doctors found their asthmatics felt better, and there were no bad effects.

Just when the allergists were comfortable prescribing antihistamines to asthmatics, Dr. Diane Schuller discovered a group of asthmatic children who got worse when they took antihistamines, thus confirming what the textbooks had been saying all along.

Did this mean that allergists were wrong and the textbooks were right? No. Dr. Schuller had merely found a small *subgroup* of asthmatic children whose asthma became worse with antihistamines. The majority of her patients tolerated antihistamines without ill effects. Furthermore, adverse reactions only occurred with certain antihistamines. So when she found that an antihistamine had caused an asthma attack, she simply switched her patient to a different antihistamine.

Helpful hint 1: If your asthma becomes worse when you use an antihistamine, throw the antihistamine into the garbage.

Helpful hint 2: If you are asthmatic and your nose is runny and itchy, you may try taking an antihistamine. You have a ninety-eight percent chance it will help you without making your asthma worse. If, perchance, the antihistamine makes your asthma worse, stop using it.

New Antihistamine Doesn't Make You Sleepy And How To Find The Best Antihistamine For You

Have you heard or read of an antihistamine that does not make you sleepy? If not, you will. Drug companies are continually searching for new chemicals. What they have discovered so far is the subject of this section.

According to the technical definition of an antihistamine, cimetadine (brand name Tagamet) is an honest-to-goodness antihistamine. However, Tagamet belongs to a completely different category of antihistamine from the ones that help allergies.

Tagamet is an anti-ulcer medicine. It stops your stomach from producing acid. Because Tagamet is so effective, it has spawned a family of antihistamines that have no drowsy side effects. However, except in very rare circumstances such as in certain cases of hives, Tagamet and the other members of that family of drugs (Ranitidine, Zantac, Pepcid) won't help allergies.

This is a case where the facts are more complicated than they might appear. You see, there are two kinds of antihistamines, called H1 and H2. The H1 kind helps allergy symptoms such as sneezing, nasal stuffiness, itchy eyes, runny nose, postnasal drainage, and hives. The H2 kind reduces stomach acid. The H1 kind can make you drowsy. The H2 kind will not. Thus, if you take Tagamet, you won't be sleepy, but you won't have much relief of your allergies either.

**How To Find An Antihistamine
That Works For Your Allergies**

Let's say you need an H1 type of antihistamine for your allergies. How do you find one that does not make you sleepy? Is there a systematic way to go about it? H1 antihistamines have such a terrible reputation it might seem useless to even try.

Luckily there is a way to find such a drug. Thanks in part to work done by Dr. Guy Settipane, doctors have a new understanding of H1 antihistamines and this understanding makes it easy to figure out which one is best for a particular individual.

First, if you read about a new drug that does not produce drowsiness, be skeptical. There are really *no* new H1 antihistamines. Instead there are four basic chemicals which clever manufacturers make into 103 brands by changing the shape, color, and name. They make tablets and capsules. They make short- and long-acting preparations. They add decongestants and aspirin. But despite these modifications there are still only *four* categories.

Some categories of antihistamines work for some people, and others work for others. Each person's body is different. You have different weight, height, muscle, fat, and metabolism. You handle medications differently. No one can predict how you will react to an antihistamine, or any other kind of drug. So the only way to find which antihistamine is best for you is to try them in a systematic way. I recommend trying one representative of each of the four categories on different days. This will *systematically* show you the one that's best for you. Do this in consultation with your doctor.

Back to the drowsy issue! When Dr. Settipane tested people for the drowsy effect, he found up to fifteen percent of people became drowsy when they used H1 antihistamines. The rest did not. So most of you can take *any* antihistamine without a problem. Others will have to experiment a little to find a suitable one. For those who cannot find an H1 antihistamine, there are other types of medication that can help.

I don't want to belabor the point, but don't automatically jump to the conclusion that you cannot take antihistamines even if you have had bad luck with several different ones. You may have been taking the same drug under a different brand name.

Some doctors may disagree with me and tell you there are more than four categories. Don't quibble. Chemists sometimes disagree about this. Humor your doctor and be willing to try a few extra pills. But if your health care professional recommends *ten* different antihistamines, you are probably wasting your time.

Ninety-five percent of over-the-counter drugs contain the identical category of antihistamine. Benadryl and Tavist are the exceptions.

You may be interested in the names of the four categories. They are ethanolamines, alkylamines, ethylenediamines, and the last category is composed of ring structures. These are technical names. You will not find them on labels. Even doctors may not be familiar with them.

Helpful hint 1: H1 antihistamines alleviate allergy symptoms, but they can cause drowsiness in about fifteen percent of people.

Helpful hint 2: The way for each of you to find the most effective antihistamine is to try a representative of each of the four categories.

Helpful hint 3: Antihistamines do not cure anybody of anything. They are for symptomatic relief. So take the least amount that controls your symptoms.

The Newest "New" Antihistamine That Doesn't Make You Sleepy

Marion Merrell Dow Company developed an antihistamine called Seldane. When it first came out, newspaper and magazine headlines proclaimed it would not make you drowsy. The drug was said to "separate sedation from relief." This is a typical example of how you must be careful of what you read.

Seldane, also called terfenadine, is a wonderful drug. However, it is not a panacea. Some people get relief and some do not. Some people get sleepy and some do not. In this respect Seldane is similar to other antihistamines.

What led newspapers to headline the non-sedating effect is a common reaction of newspapers and magazines. They isolate one fact and emphasize what is newsworthy, as opposed to what would be helpful for you to know.

When Seldane is compared to an antihistamine called Chlorpheniramine, Seldane causes less drowsiness in certain individuals. However, the company did not compare Seldane to each of the other categories of antihistamine. Limiting a comparison to one possibility out of a number of possibilities is a tried and true method to make a product seem favorable. For example, if you compare Hawaiian to Korean apples, the Hawaiian apples may taste terrific. But if you compare Hawaiian to Washington state apples, you would find Washington apples were head and shoulders above the rest.

Another aspect that newspapers failed to mention, but which the drug company was honest about, was that Seldane caused more weakness, dry mouth, and appetite increase in certain individuals than several other antihistamines.

Thus, Seldane is a wonderful drug and is definitely worth trying. But Seldane may not be the final word in antihistamine relief for *you*.

There is another factor to consider when you hear about a new drug. You must ascertain whether the drug helps you. If a drug's only redeeming value is that it doesn't make you sleepy, it will not be much use to you.

Like all drugs, Seldane has a good effect in some, a bad effect in some, and no effect in some.

Helpful hint 1: Newspaper articles tend to emphasize what editors hope will sell their papers. They do not necessarily give a balanced view.

Helpful hint 2: The only way to learn whether an antihistamine will help you is to try the antihistamine.

Helpful hint 3: The only way for you to learn whether an antihistamine will cause side effects is to try it.

Helpful hint 4: There is no perfect antihistamine that suits everyone. Each of you has a different metabolism.

Helpful hint 5: If an antihistamine does not make you sleepy but does not make you feel better either, find another antihistamine.

Non-Drowsy Or Non-Sedating

Drug companies advertise their products as non-drowsy or non-sedating. This may sound the same to you, but they are two different concepts. This is why you need to read between the lines of advertising copy.

Seldane was the first antihistamine to be developed that can be considered non-sedating. This was accomplished by altering the basic antihistamine molecule so that it could not enter the brain. Thus the drug did not slow your reflexes or interfere with your thinking process as much as traditional antihistamines, like the popular Benadryl and Chlortrimeton, which did enter the brain. Airline pilots and people working with dangerous equipment who switched to the non-sedating drugs could function normally. Two other non-sedating antihistamines are Hismanal and Claritin.

The non-sedating concept is interesting because it is like a Cinderella story where you turn a pumpkin into a coach. Chemists took an old fashioned drug, made a minor change in the molecule, and transformed it from sedating to non-sedating. Isn't chemistry wonderful?

Non-drowsy drugs, on the other hand, are not new. They are the old-fashioned decongestants like Sudafed that have been available for years. Drug companies call them non-drowsy because they can make you jittery, keep you up at night, and give you a rapid pulse. You can see why they would be called "non-drowsy".

Decongestants help you in a different way from antihistamines. Instead of drying mucus and preventing sneezing and itching, they open your nasal and sinus passages.

Helpful hint 1: Non-sedating and non-drowsy refer to the possible side effects of two different types of drugs. Non-sedating drugs don't enter the brain and don't slow your reflexes, make it difficult to think, or make you sleepy. Non-drowsy refers to decongestants which can pep you up.

Helpful hint 2: Most allergy drugs contain combinations of an antihistamine and a decongestant.

Helpful hint 3: Every medication has its advantages and disadvantages. You need to work with your doctor to figure out what is best for you.

Helpful hint 4: If you use a non-sedating drug and you are still sleepy, tell your doctor you want something else.

Helpful hint 5: If you use a non-drowsy drug that keeps you up at night or makes you jittery, tell your doctor you want something else.

Scary Seldane Side-Effect

Seldane can kill you if you take too much. So can aspirin. You can probably harm yourself with any drug if you set up the right conditions such as overuse, overdose, or use the drug in combination with certain other drugs. So it shouldn't surprise you that Seldane was eventually charged with a serious side effect even though Seldane was prescribed and loved by tens of millions of people throughout the world as the first non-sedating antihistamine.

The side effect was an irregular heartbeat that was fatal if not treated. Over a two year period twenty-five cases were reported. Two of the twenty-five died. The rest recovered. Considering the tens of millions of doses of Seldane that have been used, you have a greater chance of dying from a fatal bee-sting reaction. Nevertheless, there is no point in taking unnecessary chances.

Two antibiotics, erythromycin and ketoconazole, can increase the blood level of Seldane to undesirable levels. So can a certain antidepressant. Liver disease and advanced age can also raise the blood level.

Helpful hint 1: When a doctor prescribes a new medicine, give him a list of *all* the other medicines you use, *including* over-the-counter medicine. He can tell you if there is a potential conflict. Carry the list on a business card that fits in your wallet or purse.

A Twenty-Four Hour Antihistamine

Every year at the American Academy of Allergy and Immunology's scientific meeting doctors discuss the latest research and newest antihistamines. Some of the drugs are variations of medications that have already been approved. Some are so new they don't even have a name, merely a research number. Some fulfill their promise. Some do not.

Astemizole (brand name Hismanal) is an antihistamine that showed exceptional promise. This drug was used in Europe, Canada and Mexico for many years and proved to have a low rate of side effects. Its major advantage was that it lasted twenty-four hours in most individuals. Taking a pill once a day makes it easier to comply with the instructions.

As with many drugs there is a trade-off. Hismanal often takes three days to begin working. Many doctors don't explain this to their patients. If you are used to and want instant relief, you probably won't be happy with Hismanal.

Three other once-a-day antihistamines are loratidine (Claritin), cetirizine (Zyrtec), and ebastine.

Helpful hint 1: Once in a while doctors find truly new drugs. Hismanal (astemizole) was the first twenty-four hour, non-sedating antihistamine.

Helpful hint 2: Astemizole is only useful to *prevent* symptoms because it can take three days before it takes effect. The other once-a-day antihistamines can start working faster and may be used *either* to stop symptoms after they've started *or* to prevent them from happening.

Helpful hint 3: You may choose which way you wish to take your medicine, to stop or to prevent, but when it comes to allergy I recommend prevention. After all, an ounce of prevention can be worth a pound of cure.

Old Antihistamine Masquerades As New Antihistamine

You all know that every drug that goes into your body has a brief opportunity to do something. Then it is neutralized, destroyed, or excreted. What's interesting, at least to me, is that some drugs are active and help you when they are intact. Others help you after your body breaks the intact molecule into active fragments. Others help you after the body adds its own contribution.

Well, scientists took advantage of this situation to create a new drug from an old one. Atarax (hydroxyzine hydrochloride) is an old antihistamine. It has been available for years. After it is absorbed, it is metabolized into fragments, one of which is cetirizine.

Somewhere, a scientist woke up one morning and thought, 'Why not make cetirizine directly instead of depending on the body to make it from Atarax?'

This was done and now we have Zyrtec, a new antihistamine created from the ashes of an old antihistamine. Interestingly, cetirizine lasts twenty-four hours while Atarax lasts four. Some doctors believe cetirizine has anti-inflammatory properties in addition to being an antihistamine. If true, this is an added benefit.

Another interesting fact is that cetirizine seems stronger than Atarax. However, this may be an illusion. Cetirizine is about ten times stronger than Atarax and comes in five and ten milligram strengths. Atarax comes in ten, twenty-five and 50 fifty milligram strengths. So if you take the fifty milligram size Atarax, by the time your body metabolizes it to the active ingredient cetirizine, you will very likely have the same effect as five milligrams of cetirizine. I hope this isn't too much algebra, but the point is that cetirizine, while a good drug, isn't a miracle and, dose for dose, can probably be matched with a drug we already have.

Helpful hint 1: The doctors who figured out that making the active metabolic byproduct of Atarax were clever. This shortcuts what the body needs to do to make the drug work.

Helpful hint 2: Another drug company applied the same let's-make-an-active-metabolite-and-call-it-a-different-name logic to Seldane and created Allegra which is an active metabolite of Seldane. Its pharmacologic name is fexofenadine. Look for more active metabolites!

Six Kinds Of Adverse Drug Reactions

When the question of drug reactions comes up, it is tempting to take a shortcut and call any kind of reaction an allergic reaction without giving it any thought. However, you and your doctors must consider other possibilities. Otherwise you may get the wrong diagnosis. This kind of mistake will usually lead to incorrect treatment. There are six kinds of drug reactions.

1. Overdose

Overdose is a reaction due to taking an excess amount of a medicine or because your body accumulates too much of a medicine in your system. A child who swallows too much aspirin is an example of *taking* excess medicine. A person who has depressed liver or kidney function and therefore cannot dispose of drugs properly is an example how you can *accumulate* too much medicine in you.

2. Intolerance

Intolerance is a normal effect of a drug which is exaggerated in some individuals. For example, aspirin can cause mild irritation of the lining of your stomach. Under ordinary circumstances you won't notice this. However, certain individuals are *so* sensitive they get an ulcer and may even vomit.

3. Idiosyncrasy

Idiosyncrasy is a reaction that occurs in specific susceptible individuals. Thorazine, which is a relaxant, causes muscles to go into spasm. In susceptible individuals this can twist the body like a pretzel. It's quite uncomfortable, although it goes away if the person stops the drug.

4. Side effects

Side effects are undesirable but sometimes unavoidable responses. Decongestants and bronchodilators come from a category of drug called sympathomimetics. These open your nasal passages and your lung's airways respectively. However, they can increase your heart rate and make you jittery at the same time they are opening your respiratory passages.

5. Secondary effect

Secondary effects are indirect. Antibiotics kill bacteria that cause infection. However, they can also kill *beneficial* bacteria that reside in your intestine. This can allow *harmful* bacteria to overgrow the intestine which can lead to diarrhea or a fungus infection called candida or monilia.

6. Allergy

Allergic reactions occur from an immune response. This has nothing to do with the drug's pharmacologic action. Allergy is due to your body having made an excess amount of IgE antibody. IgE can react with drugs and cause itching, hives, asthma, and collapse.

Helpful hint 1: Most drug reactions are *not* allergic.

Helpful hint 2: If you experience anything different from usual when you take a drug, consult your doctor to find out if you are having an adverse reaction to the drug and *what kind* of adverse reaction it is.

How To Conquer Side Effects Of Drugs

Asking your doctor if a drug can cause a side effect is like asking if the sun rises in the East. Every drug can and does cause side effects in particular people.

Asking what the side effects of a drug will be will elicit a long list of possibilities. Of course, life has adverse effects, too. The real question that needs to be answered is whether a particular drug will cause side effects in *you*.

Until now no one could have told you *precisely* what are your chances of having a side effect. They would have had to give you an *average* kind of number like ten percent of the population gets this and twenty percent gets that and so on.

This is going to change! Soon we will be able to tell you exactly what will happen. At least I hope that's what we can do when we perfect our understanding of the cytochrome-P-450 enzyme system, CYP-450 for short.

CYP-450 enzymes are located in cells that primarily reside in the liver. They are responsible for breaking down drugs and getting rid of them. Otherwise one dose of a drug would stay in your body forever. CYP-450 enzymes also break down and get rid of many of the chemicals found in herbs, foods, and other substances we ingest. There are over one hundred enzymes in the CYP-450 system.

Each person has different quantities and strengths of CYP-450 enzymes. Incredibly, the activity of the enzymes can vary ten- to thirty-fold between one individual and another. You can see how this would give doctors palpitations. The same drug in the same dose can give thirty times the kick in one person than another because of how fast or slowly the CYP-450 enzymes get rid of the drug. For example, depending on your *personal* CYP-450 enzyme system a drug may last four hours or eight hours. In some cases you may metabolize the drug so fast it doesn't last two minutes!

You can see how CYP-450 enzymes can cause great discrepancy between how two people respond to the same drug.

I'd like to give you a few examples of how complicated this can be. The CYP1A2 enzyme acts on caffeine, cetirizine, theophylline, and, get ready for this you chocolate lovers, theobromine, which is a constituent of chocolate. There are several chemicals that *stimulate* CYP1A2 to work harder and several that *inhibit* CYP1A2 and make it work slower. Depending on how fast or slow your CYP1A2 works you will process the above drugs faster or slower. Thus, brocolli, brussels sprouts, and a drug called Omeprozole make the CYP1A2 enzyme work harder. Ciprofloxin and macrolide antibiotics make it work slower. Thus, taking these drugs or eating those particular foods will determine how you respond to theophylline, caffeine, cetirizine, and theobromine.

At one time there was great worry about eating grapefruit while taking Seldane. Grapefruit was said to raise the level of Seldane in the body to the point where you might suffer abnormal heart beats. What the scaremongers forgot to do was check their CYP dictionary. Grapefruit slows down the CYP2B1 enzyme. The enzyme that metabolizes Seldane is CYP3A. Not even close!

We still have a lot to learn, but this is one of the most exciting areas of *practical* research that I know of. If we can learn which enzymes do what and then learn how foods affect the enzymes, we can be much more intelligent about prescribing drugs, getting them to work better, and curing disease faster.

Helpful hint 1: One of the reasons everyone responds uniquely to medication, and even why foods affect each of us differently, resides in our CYP-450 enzyme system which breaks down drugs and foods.

Helpful hint 2: Attention chocolate lovers. Eat brocolli or brussell sprouts at the same time you eat chocolate. This will rev up your CYP1A2 enzymes which will get the chocolate out of your system faster than usual. Then you can eat more chocolate!

10

Nasal Sprays for Allergy And Sinus Symptoms

According to the Allergy and Immunology section of the National Institutes of Health in Bethesda, Maryland, over twenty-four million people in the United States suffer from nasal allergy symptoms. Since nasal sprays are efficient and convenient, many of you may have tried one of them. The chief advantage is they deliver medication directly to the nasal membrane where you need it most and where it can act fast.

The following is a description of eight types of nasal sprays that are available, how each one works, and what side effects can occur. Some of the sprays are relatively new. Others have been around for years.

Nasal Sprays For Allergy

There are old and new nasal sprays. The story is similar to the antihistamine story where some preparations are "new" because the manufacturer devised a new package for the same old ingredient and others are "new" because they are new to the United States even though they have been used in other countries for many years. Remember that "new" can mean different things to different people. The following information will give you the medical facts, and you can form your own opinion about whether the spray is new or old. My own opinion is that effectiveness and safety are more important than whether a spray is new or old.

1. Salt water

Physiologic salt water is an old-fashioned, tried and true "drug" for relieving nasal allergy symptoms. Salt water may not sound glamorous, but Dr. Sheldon Spector showed that certain patients obtain as much relief using salt water as with various drugs. The advantage of salt water is that in the proper concentration it is a natural liquid and can be used as often as you want for as long as you want.

Salt water may not work immediately, though. You should allow a trial period of one or two weeks. Two common brands are Ocean Spray and Ayr-Mist.

Helpful hint 1: Some nasal sprays are used on a one-time basis. Some sprays must be used continuously to achieve their effect. Salt-water sprays are the kind that generally need to be used continuously to achieve their effect.

2. Hot, Humid Air

Hot, humid air sounds like something your grandmother would tell you to use for nasal allergy. Grandmas often know best, but not in this case.

Dr. Robert Naclerio in Baltimore treated a group of allergic individuals with salt water steam that had been heated to thirty-seven degrees Centigrade. Although many patients reported that they felt better, Dr. Naclerio's instruments showed that their nasal stuffiness had not changed with the treatment. Higher temperatures did not increase the number of people who felt better, and there was no way to predict who would feel better and who would not.

> **Helpful hint 1**: If want to try hot, humid air for nasal symptoms, for goodness' sake don't burn yourself. These doctors used special equipment to heat and humidify the air.

> **Helpful hint 2**: Don't use hot, humid air on small children who can't tell you if the steam is burning them.

> **Helpful hint 3**: Only certain people benefit from hot, humid air.

> **Helpful hint 4**: Carrying Kleenex and an antihistamine is a lot easier than carrying a machine wherever you go so you can take hot, humid air treatments.

> **Helpful hint 5**: Some treatments seem like they are more trouble than they are worth.

3. Decongestants

Nasal decongestants shrink swollen, mucous membranes. Thus, they make it easier to breathe, sometimes help itching and sneezing, and often aid in draining your sinuses and the eustachian tube in your ear.

They work fast because they put the medicine right where you need it. Depending on the particular brand you purchase, you can obtain relief from four to twelve hours at a time.

On the other hand, nasal decongestants can produce unwanted side effects such as stinging or burning, in which case you should not use them. Another more insidious effect because you don't feel it coming on is paradoxical swelling which is called "rebound". This will make you worse. The medication first shrinks your nasal membranes but then it reacts with nasal blood vessels to make more inflammation than you had before you used the spray. Other common side effects are increased heart rate, elevated blood pressure, and jitteriness.

Don't let my warnings about stinging, burning, elevated blood pressure, and rebound scare you. These effects occur only in a small percentage of the population. Furthermore, these effects disappear when you stop using the spray. They are not long-term, permanent side effects.

So if a decongestant spray helps you and doesn't cause side effects, use it. But keep the following advice in mind. This may be common sense, but it is worth repeating.

- To determine whether a nasal decongestant elevates your blood pressure, ask your doctor to measure your blood pressure before and after you use the spray.

- If you become jittery, nervous, experience an upset stomach, or if *anything* unusual happens while you are using a decongestant (or *any* medicine for that matter), stop the medicine and consult your doctor.

- If a decongestant spray does not relieve your symptoms, stop the spray.

- If you obtain relief initially but subsequently lose the effect, stop the spray. You may be getting rebound.

- If a 12-hour spray lasts only one hour, stop the spray. This is an early warning of rebound.

- If you have symptoms other than a stuffy nose (e.g. fever, vomiting, diarrhea, earache, sore throat, cough, wheezing, anything else), stop the spray and consult your doctor.

Common decongestant sprays are:

Afrin
Coricidin Decongestant
Dristan
Duration
4-way
Neo-synephrine
NTZ
Otrivin
Privine
Sinex Decongestant

4. Antihistamine Nasal Spray

It is hard to believe that drug companies haven't put antihistamines, which are the most well-known, widely-used, and most effective medications for nasal allergy, into a nasal spray. A spray would put the antihistamine directly where it is needed.

Now Dr. Cyrille Francillon from Switzerland has tested a new antihistamine in nasal spray form and found it is effective. The medication, ebastine, has an obvious advantage. You do not have to take a pill and risk antihistamine side effects such as sleepiness which are common with oral antihistamines. Another new nasal antihistamine spray contains levocobastine.

5. Cortisone Nasal Sprays

Over the past few years, drug companies have introduced a number of cortisone nasal sprays. The companies claim that the new brands have fewer side effects and better effectiveness than the old brands. In some cases they are correct. But this is an individual matter. Each of you must try a particular spray and decide for yourself.

Cortisone sprays usually take two to three weeks just to take effect. Then you have to continue them indefinitely to maintain their effect. Many people try a few squirts and give up when they don't get instant relief. With cortisone sprays, you must be patient. Occasionally, a lucky person obtains quick relief with these sprays, but this is an exception rather than the rule.

I call cortisone nasal sprays "medicines for tomorrow" because you take them today to prevent tomorrow's problems. For *immediate* relief, you should use a decongestant or an antihistamine nasal spray.

Cortisone is an anti-inflammatory medication. Thus it is not specific for allergy. In fact, cortisone stops inflammation of *any* kind so it is also used for arthritis, burns, and certain cancers.

Be aware that cortisone nasal sprays can produce the identical dangerous side effects as cortisone pills because cortisone is absorbed into your body even when given in spray form. After a prolonged period of continual use, this can lead to the usual steroid side effects: weight gain, high blood pressure, psychological changes, cataracts in the eyes, and ulcers. In children, cortisone can stunt growth. Some nasal sprays have a greater potential for causing such side effects than others. Your allergist can discuss this with you.

Some common cortisone nasal sprays are:
Beconase
Beconase AQ
Decadron Turbinaire
Flonase
Nasacort
Nasacort AQ
Nasarel
Rhinocort
Vancenase
Vancenase AQ

6. Cromolyn Nasal Spray (Nasalcrom)

In 1967, Dr. Roger Altounyan from England discovered a drug called cromolyn. This was heralded as a wonder drug because it prevented cells in the body from releasing the chemical mediators responsible for allergic symptoms. Doctors hoped that cromolyn would be the ultimate weapon in the fight against allergy, especially since cromolyn wasn't absorbed and had no side effects.

As you might have guessed, it took awhile before cromolyn was approved for use in the United States. The name of the nasal spray is Nasalcrom. Like cortisone sprays, Nasalcrom is a "medicine for tomorrow." You usually need to use it two weeks before it takes effect. Then you must use it *continually* to *prevent* your symptoms. Unfortunately cromolyn is not perfect and won't work in all of you.

Of further interest, cromolyn was approved for use in the eyes in early 1985. The eye drops are called Crolom.

Recently, researchers looked for a better product and developed a cromolyn-like drug called Nedocromil. Technically it's a pyranoquinoline (that's a mouthful), but it works by preventing allergic reactions just like cromolyn.

7. Atropine Nasal Spray

Ipratropium Bromide is an atropine-like chemical that you inhale every four or five hours. It's most helpful for preventing a runny nose. It does not help much with sneezing or stuffy nose. The brand name is Atrovent Nasal.

8. Local Nasal Immunotherapy (LNIT)

Lastly, there is a nasal spray designed to treat the underlying cause of allergy. Researchers call this Local Nasal Immunotherapy. Doctors had hoped it would replace traditional allergy injections. LNIT is not a drug or medicine. Rather, it is a technique to immunize your nose.

With traditional allergy injections, allergists give you an injection of grass, weed, or dust to force your body to make immunity. Eventually you make enough immunity so that upon exposure to allergens, your tissues don't react.

Family doctors do the same thing when they immunize you or your children against polio and mumps. They inject the virus they don't want you to get. But they inject a *modified* form of the virus (called a vaccine), not the *really* infectious organism. This immunizes you. When the *real* polio or mumps virus comes around, your body is already protected because it has built its own immunity.

It was hoped that Local Nasal Immunotherapy would achieve the same result as allergy injections. By spraying increasing quantities of pollen into your nose, the theory was that the cells in your nose would make immunity and be protected from subsequent natural exposure.

So far LNIT has not worked well. Doctors in New York and Michigan experimented with various doses using what they call "modified" pollen. The experiment was not a glorious success. Even if LNIT had worked, the researchers only tested for ragweed and grasses. A patient who had other allergies would be out of luck. He would need traditional injections for the other allergens. Furthermore, the nasal drops were sometimes too strong and made people sneeze more.

The experiments are continuing, and you may read about them from time to time. But there is a lot more work to be done.

Helpful hint 1: There are various categories of nasal spray. Within each category, there are many different brands.

Helpful hint 2: Nasal sprays have three purposes; to stop symptoms, prevent symptoms, or force your body to build immunity. Different ingredients and techniques are required to accomplish the different goals.

Helpful hint 3: Some nasal sprays are used on a one-time basis. Some sprays must be used continuously.

Helpful hint 4: Many people think all nasal sprays are alike and do not know whether they are using cortisone, decongestants, antihistamines, saline, cromolyn, or atropine. Thus, they do not know what results to expect and therefore often misuse the sprays.

Unpleasant Side Effect Of Nasal Inhalers

We tend to think of nasal sprays as harmless. At one allergy conference Dr. Craig LaForce reported that two patients who had used a cortisone nasal spray containing beclamethasone for prolonged periods (fourteen months in one case and twenty-four in the other) perforated the cartilaginous septum in the middle of their nose. This left a hole. Other doctors have reported similar perforations with flunisolide.

Dr. LaForce thought that the combination of prolonged use and aiming the spray directly onto the nasal septum caused the perforation. But he couldn't be positive that the direction of the spray was what had caused the problem. Interestingly, one of the two patients was a nine year old child. The perforation was discovered when the child's parents reported hearing whistling sounds while the child slept. Air passing through the hole in the child's nose made the noise.

Other unpleasant side effects of cortisone nasal sprays have been reported. Dr. Julian Melamed found several patients had tightness of their chest, redness of the face, and a drop in blood pressure right after a dose of a cortisone nose spray called Flonase which has fluticasone in it. And Dr. Gerald Gleich and his colleagues reported that several patients have developed eczema around the nose from using a cortisone nose spray with budesonide in it.

Helpful hint 1: Perforation of the nasal septum, tightness of the chest, and eczema around the nose are newly recognized possible side effects of cortisone-type nasal inhalers. Fortunately these side effects are *very* uncommon.

Helpful hint 2: If you must use a nasal inhaler, don't aim it directly on your nasal septum and risk perforation.

Helpful hint 3: At various times, drug companies have tried to alleviate anxiety about the cortisone-steroid in nasal sprays by saying that cortisone-steroids don't have to be absorbed into the body to help you because they work by direct, *local* action in the nose. This is partly true. Cortisone works by its direct, local action. Then it is then absorbed into the body. By diverting your attention to where cortisone-steroids work, the companies hope you will foget what happens after the drug does its job. Unfortunately, nasal cortisone like cortisone applied anywhere in the body is *eventually* absorbed. This is like taking a small dose of cortisone-steroid each day. Over a period of time this could cause the usual side effects from prolonged use. I suppose, though, that anything is fair in the advertising game.

11

Medication and
Treatment
For Asthma

According to the National Institutes of Health over fifteen million people in the United States have asthma. This leads to loss of work, missed school, fatigue, secondary infections, and poor performance. There are also psychological problems that come from worrying and wondering when the next bad attack will occur. Severe cases of asthma result in death. There are about 5,000 deaths each year.

Asthmatics are usually surprised to learn that asthma is often due to allergy. The substances such as pollens, dust, and animals that irritate the nasal mucous membrane can irritate your lungs, too. Foods and drugs can cause asthma as well.

The following studies describe the latest findings. Because asthma is so debilitating, there is an enormous amount of research being done to combat this illness. So this section is longer than the others in this book. There are too many topics to list them in this brief preface. In general, the first group of topics tell you what asthma is, how we get it, and what effect it can have on your body. Next I wrote about the new treatments. Asthma drugs come in many shapes, forms, and sizes. Your doctors select the ones they think are best for you. However, a particular drug may not work, may cause a side effect, or may wear off over time. Each year we learn more. Each year we get smarter. In the meantime, you need to be realistic, learn what you can, and be prepared to change your treatment if something better comes along. The following studies help you keep up with the latest findings in the field of asthma treatment.

Delayed Asthma Reactions

Most asthmatics react the moment they are exposed to an allergen. In some cases, though, there is a delay of up to twelve hours. This latter type of attack is called a Late Onset or Delayed Asthma Reaction. Doctors are beginning to realize that Late Onset Reactions occur more frequently than they had thought.

Most often Late Onset Reactions occur several hours *after* an Immediate Onset Reaction. Sometimes Late Onset Reactions occur without a preceding immediate reaction.

Dr. Rami Tamir from Israel proved that Late Onset Reactions can be triggered by exposure to plant pollens. Other doctors had previously shown that they can be triggered by exposure to pets, chemicals, and foods.

Late Onset Reactions are not just a curiosity. When you develop asthma symptoms twelve hours after an exposure, it makes your diagnosis more difficult because you and your doctor may be thinking only of immediate reactions and want to blame an allergen you were exposed to at the time of the attack. Unaware that you could have reacted to a substance you were exposed to earlier in the day, you would not look into this possibility and would be condemned to repeat your mistake.

Interestingly, asthma specialists are seeing more Late Onset Reactions than they used to. This doesn't make sense when you consider that new asthma drugs are much more effective than the old ones. We are using better medicine and getting worse results.

The paradox is easy to understand. An asthmatic will usually begin coughing, wheezing, and feeling tightness of the chest when he is exposed to the substances he is allergic to. The body is not stupid and realizes it's best to leave the scene. The asthma attack is telling the person to get out of there *fast*.

However, a person who uses the highly effective medications we have these days, will take his medication and stop coughing and wheezing. This sends a message to the body that everything is under control. So instead of leaving the scene, the person stays. *Meanwhile* allergens keep assaulting the lungs and causing more and more inflammation. When the asthma medication wears off hours later, the inflammation is worse than if the person had left at the first warning. The net result is a severe attack just when the person thought he had gotten away with something.

Treatment of Late Onset Reactions

The best treatment for Late Onset Reactions is to avoid asthma-provoking allergens. When this is not possible, take medication for at least an extra twenty-four hours after an immediate-onset attack. If you discontinue too soon, you may be trapped and it will be too late for you to escape from a severe attack.

Helpful hint 1: Thanks to research, doctors are aware of Late Onset Reactions. Understanding these reactions has helped us treat what had been many puzzling and difficult cases.

Helpful hint 2: If you experience Late Onset Reactions, take your medication from twelve to twenty-four hours after exposure even though you have no symptoms.

Helpful hint 3: You can suffer from delayed nasal and eye allergy symptoms, too.

Helpful hint 4: Sometimes modern medicine can backfire by preventing your symptoms so effectively that you are unaware you are exposing yourself to harmful allergens.

Sinus Infections Can Cause Asthma

If you have sinus disease and asthma, you will be encouraged by the research of Dr. Ray Slavin. Dr. Slavin is a well-thought-of doctor who gets the toughest cases. Many of his patients need high doses of steroids. Fortunately for his patients, Dr. Slavin is a doctor who keeps looking for ways to help his patients. With his never-give-up attitude he treated certain patients who had sinus disease complicating their asthma, and he found that when he got rid of their sinus disease their asthma improved. He didn't cure their asthma, but he was able to reduce the amount of steroids these patients needed. And reducing the need for steroids is always a significant achievement.

Keep in mind that many patients who claim they have sinus disease do not have sinus disease. Furthermore, not all asthmatics in Dr. Slavin's study improved. Nevertheless the ones who did improve were so much better that this is worth looking into. Even if stopping your sinus disease doesn't help your asthma, at least your sinuses feel better.

Helpful hint 1: If you have asthma and sinus disease, ask your doctor to treat your sinus problem vigorously. This may help your asthma.

Risk Of Developing Asthma In Occupations Where There Is Exposure To Animals

People who work in pet stores, research laboratories, and veterinary offices are heavily exposed to various animals. Many of them are properly concerned that prolonged exposure might sensitize them and result in asthma. Those who are constantly exposed to pets in their homes should be concerned too, but like most of my patients they probably don't want to think that they might become sensitized.

Dr. Richard Evans studied how and when asthma began in 400 laboratory workers. He found that the individuals who became allergic had a history of allergy as children, had converted to a positive skin test to the animals they worked with, and showed a lung reaction when they breathed a drug called methacholine which is a test to detect the kind of hyperreactive airways that are characteristic of asthma.

On average, Dr. Evans' patients developed asthma from four months to two years after they had begun working with the animals.

Helpful hint 1: Risk factors for developing asthma to animals include a history of allergy as a child, an asthmatic response to a test called methacholine challenge, and a positive skin test to the animal.

Helpful hint 2: After four years of exposure, only four of the 400 patients Dr. Evans studied had developed asthma. So the risk of asthma is not great. And you should not be overly paranoid about exposure to animals.

Helpful hint 3: On the other hand, if you have already developed allergy to animals, at home or at work, you *should be* overly paranoid. It is your duty to yourself to avoid animals you are allergic to.

Helpful hint 4: Denying that you might become allergic to a pet because you are not currently allergic to a pet is a helpful way to avoid reality.

Asthma-Provoking Chemical Found In Medicine Used To Treat Asthma

The alarming discovery that there is a chemical in certain anti-asthma medicines that can trigger asthma is a situation where the cure turns out to be worse than the disease. In this case, the cure *causes* the disease.

I don't know if you have read much about sulfites. They are chemical preservatives that are used to keep vegetables fresh, especially in salad bars. But sulfites aren't restricted to salad bars. They are used to preserve medications, too. Like many good things, though, sulfites have their downside.

Asthmatics who need to use a mechanical respirator to inhale their medication are at risk for this sort of problem. At the time of use, they pour the drug into the respirator, thus exposing the drug to air. Manufacturers need to add a preservative to protect the drug's potency during the pouring step. The preservative they use is often the same bisulfite that is used on vegetables. Thus asthmatics who are sulfite-sensitive risk aggravating their asthma when they use mechanical nebulizers.

The phenomenon is called Paradoxical Asthma because the active ingredient makes you feel better, yet the preservative accompanying the active ingredient makes you feel worse!

Don't panic. This only applies to the bronchodilator solutions that are used in the motor-driven nebulizers. The common hand-held pressurized cannisters don't need this chemical since the solutions in them are not exposed to air. Fortunately (and this is a lucky circumstance) only a few people react to the preservative. So most of you can use what are called nebulized drugs without difficulty. However, if you use a nebulizer and become worse after treatment, tell your doctor right away.

Hopefully, by the time you read this most drug companies will have replaced the sulfites with something safer.

Helpful hint 1: If you take any medication or treatment and notice your allergic symptoms become worse or if you experience side effects, stop the drug and consult your doctor.

Tylenol Provokes Asthma

If you have asthma and thought you just had to worry about sulfites in addition to dogs, cats, and pollens, you are wrong. Dr. R. Settipane found that high doses of Tylenol (acetaminophen) can trigger asthma, too. Tylenol is one of a dozen or so non-steroidal anti-inflammatory drugs. All except acetaminophen had been know to cause asthma, so doctors felt they could prescribe Tylenol to their sensitive asthmatics with impunity. Now we have to be more careful because even acetaminophen can provoke asthma.

The good news is that acetaminophen-sensitivity is exceedingly rare, and when it occurs it is easy to treat.

Helpful hint 1: Non-steroidal anti-inflammatory drugs can cause asthma. The common ones are aspirin, Naprosyn, Alleve, Ibuprofen, and Motrin. By the time you read this book there will be other brands.

Helpful hint 2: When your doctor prescribes a medicine or even if you take an over-the-counter preparation, ask your doctor whether the new drug conflicts with a drug you are already taking.

Sudden Fatal Asthma With Open Airways

How can you have fatal asthma with *open* airways when, by definition, your airways are *closed* during an asthma attack?

To be honest, I don't know the answer.

Dr. Richard Nicklas reported he had found a group of asthmatics who were using asthma drugs called beta-agonist bronchodilators. Although these drugs are effective in opening your airways, they can have a side effect of initiating an abnormal heart rhythm. The abnormal heartbeat can be severe enough to lead to cardiac arrest.

Interestingly, the fatalities Dr. Nicklas reported did *not occur* while these patients were in the *midst* of an asthma attack. Although these people had underlying asthma, at the time of their death their bronchial tubes were wide open *and* they were not having trouble breathing. Hence the fatality occurred "with open airways" since the death was actually due to cardiac arrest.

Despite the fact that the deaths occurred when there were no asthma symptoms, doctors named this condition Fatal Asthma. I don't know why the doctors chose this name. To me, 'Fatal Heart Arrhythmia Disease' would be more appropriate.

So far these deaths have only occurred in people who use excessive levels of beta agonists or in certain elderly people who cannot excrete these drugs quickly, thus causing the drug to accumulate in their system to toxic levels.

Helpful hint 1: Doctors sometimes attach strange names to diseases that tell you nothing about the disease or its underlying cause.

Helpful hint 2: Excessive levels of *any* drug, including vitamins and aspirin, can be dangerous. Be careful!

Asthma-Mimic Found In The Stomach

No allergist worth his degree wants to be caught treating asthma when the problem is due to an asthma-mimic. So allergists look for asthma-mimics everywhere. Believe it or not, the most recent sighting has been in the stomach.

Gastroesophageal reflux is the scientific name for what causes acid indigestion. Stomach acid is supposed to stay in the stomach where it belongs. However, the valves and muscles that keep the acid there are sometimes weak. This allows acid to back up into the esophagus which is the tube leading from your mouth to your stomach. Acid-backup causes sour taste in the mouth, belching, hoarseness, cough, and chest pain. Millions of Americans take tons of antacids to relieve these kinds of symptoms.

Dr. Richard Irwin who is at the University of Massachusetts Medical School found that it is easy for doctors and patients to be fooled into thinking allergy and asthma when they should be thinking acid reflux and indigestion. Acid in the esophagus can cause a chronic cough that mimics asthma. The cough is persistent, worse at night, and often occurs after meals.

Complicating the picture is the fallacy that a person can have only one disease at a time. Many patients who have true asthma are made worse by acid reflux. These people need treatment for asthma *and* acid-reflux simultaneously.

Helpful hint 1: If you cough when you lie down or after heavy meals, you may have acid-reflux and not asthma.

Helpful hint 2: If you have asthma and your asthma is worse at night, upon lying down, or after heavy meals, acid-reflux may be complicating your asthma.

Helpful hint 3: You have nothing to lose by asking your doctor to check you for acid-reflux. If you want to impress your doctor, say you want to be tested for gastroesophageal reflux, but practice this a few times in front of a mirror so you don't stumble over the words.

You May Not Have Asthma

As you just read, other diseases can mimic asthma. Because you have difficulty breathing, coughing, wheezing, and tightness of the chest does not mean you have asthma. Your doctors need to take a careful history, examine you, and do testing to know for sure.

Dr. Ellen Garibaldi from St. Louis described a woman who had breathlessness, wheezing, and cough during exercise. This is considered a sure sign of exercise-induced asthma. The woman even had a lung function test that indicated asthma. However, when the woman did not respond to asthma treatment, Dr. Garibaldi was smart enough to re-examine her.

Using a very special technique called videostroboscopic laryngoscopy, she videotaped the woman's vocal cords while the woman was exercising and found the vocal cords closed when they should have been open. This narrowed the woman's airway and made it difficult to breathe.

To make sure she wasn't being fooled by another condition, Dr. Garibaldi put a paralyzing material on her patient's vocal cords. With the vocal cords paralyzed so they couldn't close, the woman had no problem during exercise. She couldn't talk, but she could run to her heart's content.

Other asthma-mimics are the anti-depressant, Prozac, and certain antihypertensive drugs like Vasotec.

Helpful hint 1: Asthma is a specific reaction that takes place in the small airways of the lung. This causes coughing, wheezing, tightness of the chest, and difficulty breathing. Unfortunately other conditions and certain medications can cause the same symptoms, so diagnosis can be challenging.

Helpful hint 2: If you are being treated for asthma and your treatment is not working as you would like, consider the possibility that your diagnosis is not correct.

Overdiagnosis And Overtreatment Of Black Asthmatics

In order to diagnose asthma, some doctors rely quite heavily on lung function tests. As you would expect, they compare their patient's lung function to a normal standard. If their patient's test result is below normal, the doctors conclude that their patient has asthma.

What would happen if the normal values were wrong? The answer: Doctors would make the wrong diagnosis.

This happened to several patients who were treated at Meharry Medical College. Two astute doctors realized that their clinic had been using a standard that was based on a group of White asthmatics. When the doctors investigated more thoroughly, they learned that Blacks have a different set of normal values. With this information, they reviewed their patients and identified those who had been diagnosed asthmatic but who were actually not asthmatic.

The lung function test can also be used to decide how much asthma medicine an asthmatic should take. The more abnormal the test, the more medicine the patient requires. Thus if a Black person's dose was based on incorrect values, the person would be taking more medicine than necessary.

I don't want to leave the impression there has been widespread misdiagnosis and overtreatment. These cases involved only a few patients because doctors don't usually rely *solely* on lung function tests to make a diagnosis of asthma. Ordinarily they coordinate the lung function test with a thorough history, the right questions, a good physical examination, and allergy skin tests.

Helpful hint 1: If you are Black and were diagnosed asthmatic *solely* on the basis of a lung function test, ask your doctor to double check your situation.

Discovery Of What Provokes Asthma After Exercise

Exercise triggers asthma in many patients. Because up to ten percent of people have this problem, Drs. Regis McFadden and Sandra Anderson studied the condition hoping to learn how to treat other types of asthma. They examined oxygen, carbon dioxide, sugar, and hormone levels. They reasoned that these substances change during exercise and therefore must be responsible for the symptoms.

As sometimes happens, this approach led nowhere. So the doctors took a different approach and examined the effect on the lungs of cooling and water loss during heavy exercise.

In Dr. McFadden's case, he found his patients experienced bronchospasm due to *cooling* of the lungs. When you exercise, you breathe faster to cool down and dissipate the extra body heat. The identical reaction occurs when cold air hits your lungs, which, obviously, cools your lungs.

Dr. Anderson, who performed her research in Australia, found *her* patients experienced exercise-induced asthma due to *loss of water* as they breathed faster and faster, not because their lungs were cooling off.

Interestingly you can prevent exercise-induced asthma by using a device that warms the air as it enters your lungs or by altering the humidity of the inhaled air. Any of you who have exercise-induced wheezing may have noticed that running activities invariably trigger wheezing while swimming with your face in the water (high humidity) does not.

Helpful hint 1: Depending on the particular patient, exercise-induced wheezing is due to the rate of cooling or the rapid loss of water from the lungs.

Helpful hint 2: Exercise-induced wheezing is a specific entity and refers only to wheezing that occurs *after* exercise stops. Wheezing that begins *during* exercise is not generally considered to be the exercise kind.

Helpful hint 3: Sometimes scientists investigate a disease and uncover changes that have taken place such as the chemical changes that take place during vigorous exercise. But the changes are not responsible for the disease. Instead these changes are labelled "associated findings" to emphasize the fact that they do not indicate a cause-and-effect relationship.

Exercise-Induced Asthma Is Unrecognized

Dr. L. Kalish from Georgia examined exercise-induced asthma in high school athletes. Thirteen percent of the teenagers were found to have this condition. Although this seems like a high figure, other studies have shown comparable prevalence in other groups of people. For example, Dr. Henry Dold of Illinois reported about 8 percent of the 1988 United States Olympic team had exercise-induced asthma.

As I mentioned previously, exercise-induced asthma produces wheezing, coughing, and tightness of the chest shortly *after* you exercise. If your symptoms occur *during* exercise, this is *not* exercise-induced asthma.

These findings are important because many children are undiagnosed and may be performing below their capability. However, when making this diagnosis, your doctors must be careful they aren't just dealing with lack of conditioning.

Helpful hint 1: Exercise-induced asthma has been found to occur in more children than previously thought.

Helpful hint 2: Exercise-induced asthma does not prevent outstanding achievement in sports. Many asthmatics become Olympic athletes despite this condition.

Asthma Worse If Family Member Smokes

Smoking can cause health problems for the person who smokes. It is now apparent that people who are merely exposed to cigarette smoke can suffer too.

Dr. Andrew Murray reported that asthmatic children who are exposed to their parents' cigarette smoke have more symptoms than those who live in homes where neither parent smokes. The effect was strongest in closed, poorly ventilated rooms which is typical in winter months when the windows are likely to be closed and children are likely to be playing indoors.

In previous studies doctors had noted the same sort of effect in offices where people work in a closed environment.

Helpful hint 1: No one has shown that smoking is beneficial to your health.

Helpful hint 2: For your own health and for the health of others, it is best to stop smoking.

Peak-Flow Meters

Prescribing peak-flow meters has become a hot treatment in allergy. I can hardly think of any doctor or respiratory therapist who does not approve and strongly recommend their use.

Blow into the device, and you get a reading of how your lung function compares to the normal value for someone of your age and size. By keeping a daily diary and comparing your result to what is expected, you can monitor your asthma.

Peak flow meters are used in the home to give you an early warning of when you are getting worse and alert you to *raise* your dose of medication before it's too late. This can prevent an emergency dash to the hospital.

On the other hand, if your peak-flow diary shows your lung function is normal for several days in a row, you can do the reverse. You can *reduce* your medication. Consult your doctor first, but steady, normal readings often indicate a crisis has passed and you can reduce your medication without harm.

Peak-flow meters are also used in doctors' offices to determine whether you can have your allergy immunizing injection that day. The assumption is that if your lung function is not normal, the added allergen in the injection might trigger an acute attack. If your lung function is normal, the injection would be tolerated.

The assumption that peak-flow can give advance warning of how you will tolerate an allergy injection, while perfectly reasonable, was tossed out the window by an inquisitive nurse, J. M. Dunn.

Ms. Dunn had the bright idea to double check the prevailing assumption and find out for herself whether peak flow predicted what would happen. She discovered that a peak flow done just before administration of an allergy immunizing injection did not predict how a patient would tolerate his injection. Some patients reacted even though their peak flow measured in the normal range, and others did not react even though their peak flow was reduced below normal.

According to Ms. Dunn, the most accurate predictor, and even this wasn't one hundred percent, was a history taken in the office by an allergist who had experience treating allergic asthma.

Another disagreeable report, disagreeable to allergists because it challenges our ideas, came from Dr. Andre Cartier who practices in Quebec, Canada. He and his associates gave patients peak-flow meters and asked the patients to keep diaries of their progress. Unknown to the patients, the meters had electronic memories.

When the patients showed up with their hand-written diaries, the doctors compared the diaries to the electronic record. Nearly twenty percent of the patients wrote phony numbers so they wouldn't disappoint their doctors. Another group didn't use the meters and didn't write anything. These latter people evidently didn't care what their doctors thought about their not being compliant and made no effort to hide their non-compliance.

Do You Need A Peak-Flow Meter?

Discuss whether you need a peak-flow meter with your doctor. Keep in mind, however, that coughing, wheezing, tightness of the chest, wheezing during exercise, or waking up at night with coughing means your peak flow is down and you need medicine. This is common sense.

On the other hand you may want a peak flow meter to monitor a child. But a child who is coughing, short of breath, getting up at night, and so forth needs medicine no matter what the peak flow meter says.

The moral is this: When you have asthma, *you have to pay attention to your body*. If you do not want to be bothered thinking about what is happening to you, you should use a peak-flow meter.

Helpful hint 1: If you are coughing, wheezing, having tightness of the chest, or waking up at night with asthma, you don't need a peak flow meter to tell you something is wrong. However, if you like to have a number to tell you how miserable you are, buy and use a peak-flow meter.

Helpful hint 2: Several studies have shown that one third of patients don't use their peak flow meters.

Helpful hint 3: Some patients want to please their doctors so much they will falsify data and pretend they have done what they are supposed to do rather than be honest with their doctor and give him a chance to figure out another way to help them.

Helpful hint 4: We ought to have an award for nurses like J. Dunn who don't assume that standard operating procedure is correct and take the trouble to double-check what we are doing. She had the brilliance to question a standard dogma and uncover the truth.

Vomiting And Nausea From Asthma Medicines

This report is a classic example of how drugs can react with each other and make you ill. It is a good reminder to be careful when mixing medications. In technical terms this is called drug-drug interaction, and there is a huge book, *Drug Interactions-Facts and Comparisons* by David Tatro from Stanford University that documents all the drug interactions we know about.

Cephalosporins are antibiotics which are related to penicillin. Since they do not cause as many allergic reactions as penicillin, they are safer to use. From the time of their inception, the drug industry has improved upon them by creating newer, stronger, and more stable compounds. This report is about the third generation of cephalosporins.

Four of the third generation cephalosporins can create a special problem for allergy sufferers. When your body metabolizes these four (see below), it breaks them into pieces, one of which happens to be disulfiram or Antabuse. You may have heard of Antabuse. This drug is prescribed to prevent alcoholics from drinking. When taken with alcohol, Antabuse produces flushing, throbbing headaches, vomiting, chest pain, weakness, and confusion. This is a powerful deterrent to drinking alcohol.

Unfortunately, certain allergy preparations, such as antihistamines, cold remedies, and theophylline, can contain up to twelve percent alcohol when dispensed in liquid form. Thus, if you are taking any of the four cephalosporins, you will have Antabuse in your bloodstream as the cephalosporin is metabolized. If at the same time you use one of the liquid preparations containing alcohol, you may experience the alcohol-Antabuse reaction. This won't be fun.

The four cephalosporins are cefamandole (Mandol), cefoperazone (Cefobid), cefuroxime (Zinacef, Kefurox), and moxalactan (Moxam). There will undoubtedly be more brands of third generation cephalosporins as drug companies do more research, so consult your doctor.

Helpful hint 1: Mixing drugs is not a good idea unless you know what you are doing.

Helpful hint 2: Certain cephalosporins are broken down into an Antabuse-like chemical.

Beta Blockers Can Make Asthma Worse

Beta blockers are prescribed for angina, hypertension, glaucoma, and even migraine headache. Some people use beta blockers to calm themselves before giving public presentations. Common beta blockers are Inderal, Corgard, Blocadren, Lopressor, Tenormin, and Timoptic.

In certain individuals beta blockers are a two-edged sword. Although effective for cardiac and vascular conditions, they can exacerbate allergies.

Dr. John Toogood from Canada reported that certain patients who take beta blockers experience heightened allergic reactions to foods, certain drugs, insect stings, and X-ray contrast material. Although allergy injections don't contain drugs, beta blockers can increase reactions to allergy injections as well.

These findings do not mean you must stop using beta blockers. They merely mean you must be alert to the possibility that this drug can backfire. So be prepared to switch to another type of drug if you experience adverse effects when a doctor prescribes a beta blocker for you.

Helpful hint 1: If you are using drugs and notice new or different symptoms, consider the possibility that the drugs are responsible for the change in your condition.

Long-Lasting Inhaler For Asthma

At a company called Winthrop-Breon, researchers found a way to make metered dose asthma inhalers last longer than the usual four hours. The chemical they invented is bitolterol mesylate. The brand name is Tornalate.

Bitolterol mesylate is actually inactive. But when you inhale it, one of your lung's enzymes breaks it into small molecules. One of these smaller molecules is a chemical called colterol. Colterol is an *active* drug and belongs to the epinephrine family in which are several of the most powerful anti-asthma drugs available.

Since it takes time for the lung's enzymes to convert the bitolterol mesylate to the active ingredient colterol, this inhaler can last up to eight hours. Unfortunately, in some people, the lung's enzymes work twice as hard so bitolterol mesylate only lasts four hours, the same as most inhaled bronchodilator drugs.

Now we have other long-lasting inhalers, salmeterol (Serevent) and formoterol. Salmeterol does not depend on your lung's enzymes. Instead it is a long, stretched-out molecule. Since its duration of action is independent of your body's enzymes, it is more reliable for a long-lasting effect. Serevent can last up to twelve hours.

Helpful hint 1: A clever scientist can alter a drug so that the drug helps you for a prolonged period of time.

Helpful hint 2: In the case of Tornalate the body can outwit the smartest scientist and ruin the best intentions.

Helpful hint 3: If you use an inhaled bronchodilator, you may want to try the long-acting kind. They might reduce the frequency with which you must use your inhaler and make it easier for you to control your asthma.

Right- and Left-Handed Drugs?

Did you know that many drugs are right and left handed? This sounds like a trick question from a practical joker, but it's a fact of life.

The currently-used bronchodilator tablets for asthma are called chiral molecules. This means they are shaped with right and left spirals. Each pill has equal amounts of right- and left-handed molecules.

Interestingly left-handed molecules are the more effective ones in the human body. In fact studies show that the right-handed ones can make asthma worse.

In a cruel twist of fate the body seems to get rid of the good, left-handed molecules first, leaving the right-handed ones behind. So some allergists have worried that our current crop of bronchodilators may make certain people worse.

Scientists are now trying to test this theory. Hopefully they will have the answer soon. In the meantime, keep taking your medicine if it helps you.

Helpful hint 1: The human body is extraordinarily resilient. Don't let philosophical arguments by a group of nervous nellies debating the theoretical implications of right- and left-handed molecules stop you from using medicine that clearly helps you.

Helpful hint 2: If you find you are getting worse while taking bronchodilators, consult your doctor. You may be one of the rare individuals where right- and left-handed molecules make a difference.

Albuterol Powder And Ketotifen--Two New Drugs For Asthma

Albuterol powder and Ketotifen tablets are new and exciting asthma drugs.

1. Albuterol Powder

Albuterol is perhaps the most common medication prescribed for asthma. It produces fast, efficient relief. For the most part it comes in two forms, tablets and inhalers.

The advantage of tablets is that they get into your body without any effort except learning how to swallow a pill. There are two disadvantages. It takes time for the drug to reach your lungs, and on the way to the lungs albuterol can cause nervousness, rapid heart beat, and elevated blood pressure. With an inhaler, albuterol goes right where it's needed, works fast, and bypasses the rest of your body where side effects could occur. The disadvantage is that it takes expert coordination to use an inhaler *properly*. While you are coughing, wheezing, and gasping for breath, you must remember to shake the cannister, exhale, activate the cannister, and inhale at *precisely* the right moment. Otherwise, the drug does not penetrate deeply and does no good.

To make inhaling easier and thus enable albuterol to work more effectively, a drug company developed albuterol *powder*. The brand is Rotocap, and at a recent scientific meeting of the American Academy of Allergy, Dr. James Kemp explained why albuterol powder is better than the traditional, pressurized, liquid metered-dose inhaler.

To use the Rotahaler, which is the name of the device that delivers the powder to your lungs, you place a capsule in the bottom of a two-chambered container about the size of a policeman's whistle. Twist the container. This breaks the capsule and spills the powder into the bottom of the container. Then you suck on the top part of the container. Since your breath sucks the powder out of the cannister, the the result is a more effective and wider distribution of the drug onto the surface of your lungs than if you rely on a propellant to do the job.

2. Ketotifen

In the early 1970's a drug company in England developed cromolyn. This was the first *anti-allergy* drug. It stabilized certain cells in the body so the cells could not release chemical mediators, like histamine, which as you learned earlier are the chemicals that are *directly* responsible for allergic symptoms. Other allergy drugs fought off the chemical mediators *after* they had been released from their cells. Cromolyn was able to *prevent release* of chemical mediators in the first place.

The problem with cromolyn is that the body doesn't absorb it so you have to spray the drug whereever you need it, in your eyes, nose, lungs, or all three locations, depending on where you have symptoms. Three sprays at a time is a lot of spraying. Wouldn't it be nice if drug companies could alter cromolyn so your body could absorb it so one dose could travel to *all* parts of you and do the work of three sprays?

Well, lo and behold, the drug companies went to work and twenty-five years later we have Ketotifen which, like cromolyn, can *prevent* allergy reactions. Unlike cromolyn, though, Ketotifen can be absorbed.

As with any drugs, Albuterol Powder and Ketotifen tablets help certain individuals and not others.

Helpful hint 1: Sometimes a drug is "new" simply because doctors learn more efficient and more effective ways to deliver it to affected parts of your body.

Helpful hint 2: New does not necessarily mean the drug is better for you. You must try it to find out.

Whether To Use or Not To Use Your Inhaler-- That Is the Question!

Dr. Malcolm Sears from New Zealand caused consternation in the allergy community when he reported that chronic, everyday use of inhaled bronchodilators caused an increased number of asthmatic deaths. No one disagrees that overusing inhalers can cause death. This had actually been known since the late 1970's when doctors in England traced an increased number of deaths to an isuprel inhaler that was sold in Great Britain and contained a double-dose of medication. What allergists hadn't agreed on and still don't agree on is, "What is overuse?"

Dr. Sears and many advisors to the National Institutes of Health say inhalers should only be used to rescue you from sudden unexpected attacks. Others say that chronic use is all right as long as you don't exceed a certain limit.

In other words the answer to how often to use an inhaler depends on when, how severe, and under what circumstances your symptoms occur. It depends on whether you have other medical conditions, what you're allergic to, and whether you're using other medicine.

Helpful hint 1: Don't be swayed by sweeping generalizations of the medical profession. Consult your doctor and find out what is best for you.

Whether You'll Have or Not Have Your Inhaler To Use?, That Is the Other Question

In 1987 the industrialized nations met in Montreal and agreed on the Montreal Protocol. The purpose was to ban fluorocarbon production by the year 1996 to protect the ozone layer because fluorocarbons deplete ozone.

The problem is that fluorocarbon is the propellant in most metered-dose, asthma inhalers.

Drug companies have had to rush to come up with an alternative. So far the best hope is a device invented in Scandinavia called Turbuhaler. Now there is a second device called Pulvinal. These two multi-dose-containing devices are filled with powder but can deliver a *single* dose of powder with each breath.

There are other powder-containing devices where you have to load a single dose each time. These are called Rotahaler, which was described above, and Diskhaler.

What is exciting about Turbuhaler is that when used properly Turbuhaler delivers twenty percent of the medication to your lungs. The standard inhalers we all know and love, the ones where fluorocarbons are the propellant, deliver about ten percent of the medication to the lungs.

Helpful hint 1: Although inhalers with fluorocarbon propellants may be phased out, medical science already has a good substitute.

Helpful hint 2: It is shocking to learn that even when you use proper inhalation technique, only ten to twenty percent of the drug gets to the lungs where it is needed.

Helpful hint 3: These new, non-propellant inhalers may be useless if you don't have proper instruction. With fluorocarbon-propellant inhalers, you had to breathe slow and steady. With the new powder inhalers, you must breathe quick and fast because *you* are the propellant and you have to create enough force to get the drug into your lungs.

Anti-inflammatory Drugs (Cortisones) Are The Hot Treatment for Asthma

Asthma is due to tightening of the muscles on the *outside* surface of your bronchial airways, allergic inflammation and secondary infection which occurs *inside* your airways, and activation of certain nerve fibers *within* the airway wall. On the next page is a diagram that shows where the pathology occurs and, in parentheses, the type of medication that can correct the pathology.

Because of the multiple causes, an asthmatic often needs several medications depending on which pathology seems most likely responsible. This varies from one person to another.

What has happened over the past few years, however, is that doctors have focused their attention on inflammation and ignored the other components of the asthmatic reaction, sometimes even when a patient is already getting good results with a traditional bronchodilator.

The trend is so strong that many doctors don't advocate bronchodilators at all, just anti-inflammatory drugs. This means cortisone is being recommended more often and at all ages, even in children. You can read about this in the national guidelines for treating asthma that have been published by the National Institutes of Health in Bethesda, Maryland.

Muscle constriction   Nerve endings
   (bronchodilator)   (anti-cholinergic)

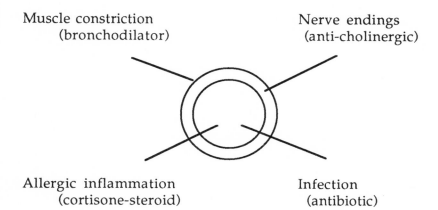

Allergic inflammation   Infection
   (cortisone-steroid)   (antibiotic)

Antibiotics get rid of infection.
Bronchodilators relax the constricted muscle.
Anti-cholinergics work on the nerve endings.
Cortisone-steroids help the inflammation.

On the other hand, anti-inflammatory drugs like the cortisone-steroids can have serious and permanent side effects. When used regularly they can cause cataracts in the eyes, osteoporosis (thinning of the bones), weight gain, diabetes, and emotional reactions. So, why the switch from bronchodilators which have no long-term side effects to cortisone-steroids that are known to cause long-term side effects?

Although there are very few diseases where one treatment works in every case, doctors never give up hoping to find a sure-cure. In the case of asthma many doctors think cortisone-steroid is the ultimate anti-asthma drug. They came to this conclusion because certain asthmatics who did not respond to bronchodilator-type drugs, which were the treatment of choice at one point in time, responded to cortisone-steroids. So cortisone-steroids became the new treatment of choice.

Of course, eventually doctors found patients who didn't respond to cortisone-steroids or who only responded to such high doses that they quickly gained weight, fractured bones from osteoporosis, and developed cataracts. Ordinarily this would have sent doctors in search of *another* treatment of choice. But in the case of cortisone-steroids, thinking seems to have stagnated and all I can tell you is that many professors advocate cortisone-steroids as the first and only type of drug to be used in every asthmatic.

There are several new and exciting non-cortisone anti-inflammatory and anti-chemical-mediator drugs being studied, but so far none of them have fulfilled their promise of alleviating *difficult* cases of asthma the way cortisone-steroids can.

What is puzzling is that doctors have always known that steroids were helpful for asthma, but they were somewhat reluctant to prescribe them until other, safer methods, like bronchodilators or getting rid of the cat, had been tried. Now, many physicians advocate steroids from the beginning. If you want to know why, you'll have to ask them. I don't understand this.

Helpful hint 1: Although many physicians, including some from the prestigious National Institutes of Health, recommend steroids as the first and only drug to prescribe for asthma, steroids can have permanent and serious side effects. You should try safer methods first. Of course, if safer methods don't help, you have no choice but to take cortisone-steroids.

Spacers For Asthma Inhalers

Bronchodilator-containing inhalers are fast-acting, but studies show that only ten to fifteen percent of the drug reaches your lungs even when you use the proper inhalation technique.

To make inhalers more efficient, doctors tried placing a tube, like the cardboard inside a roll of toilet paper, between the inhaler and the mouth. This is called a spacer. There are many different brands, and some inhalers come with a spacer permanently attached.

When you activate the inhaler, the drug passes through the tube, through your mouth, and into your lungs. The result is better distribution of the medication in your lungs. This translates into better relief.

Unfortunately, many patients think a spacer works like a reservoir to hold the drug. They think that it isn't important where they aim the inhaler or how they time their breathing. They think they can be casual and aim the device whichever way they want as long as it is in the general direction of their lungs.

Dr. Jerry Dolovich showed that proper inhaler-technique is *more* critical with a spacer than without because you have to overcome the tendency to be sloppy because you think the spacer does the work for you.

If you pause in your inhalation when you use a spacer, up to eighty percent of the drug lands on the inside of the tube. Only twenty percent reaches the mouth. And from other studies that show how much is lost on the way between the mouth and the lungs, you could end up with *only two percent* of the drug going into your lungs.

In a real-life study, Dr. John Toogood, who has a passion for practicality, did an experiment to see if spacers lived up to their promise. He found that half of the patients who used one achieved better relief. Half did not. His conclusion about how to tell which patients would benefit and which would not? What do you think? Trial and error is the correct answer.

Helpful hint 1: For certain asthmatics a "spacer" increases the effectiveness of inhaled bronchodilator medicine. This means better relief.

Helpful hint 2: If you are not obtaining satisfactory relief using an inhaler, try a spacer.

Helpful hint 3: When you swallow a pill, you know it is in you. When you use a spacer, any number of things can go wrong to prevent you from getting the full effect of the medicine.

Helpful hint 4: If you use a spacer, you must inhale and *keep inhaling* as you activate the inhaler. Failure to do so results in up to eighty percent loss of the drug in the spacer's tube and valve, another eighteen percent loss in the mouth and throat, and only two percent reaching your lungs.

Helpful hint 5: Because spacers can be difficult to use properly, many people will not benefit from this new development.

Helpful hint 6: A treatment that is new does not necessarily benefit everyone who tries it.

Spacers for Cortisone-Steroid Inhalers

Spacers for cortisone-steroid inhalers came about after doctors discovered how spacers made inhaled bronchodilators more effective. Seeing that certain asthmatics needed less *total* medication as a result of using a spacer, they hoped that patients who inhaled their cortisone-steroid would be able to reduce their *total* dose of cortisone-steroid since the drug went directly into the lungs where it was needed.

Guess what? Cortisone-steroid inhalers worked. They worked so well that doctors prescribed them for thousands of asthmatics. With increased use, side effects cropped up. The most common side effects were yeast infections in the mouth called candidiasis, irritation of the throat, and hoarseness due to steroid landing on the vocal cords as the cortisone-steroid passed through on its way to the lungs.

Dr. Les Hendeles, who is a pharmacologist, reported that spacers can prevent these side effects. He also found spacers can prevent the momentary cough some people experience when they inhale steroids.

Helpful hint 1: When doctors discover a new technique, like using a spacer to improve the efficiency of delivering medication to the lungs, they get excited and try to apply the technique to other situations. In this case adding a spacer to cortisone inhalers helped many patients avoid cortisone-steroid side effects in their oral cavity.

Helpful hint 2: Another way to reduce the chance of a candida infection from cortisone-steroid inhalers is rinse your mouth after you use your inhaler.

Theophylline As The New Wonder Drug

No one seems to like theophylline any longer. It used to be the darling of asthma doctors. Study after study showed how well it worked and how it saved lives.

Suddenly theophylline became the most vilified drug in the pharmacy. It didn't work. It caused too many side effects. It was outdated. And so on.

The problem is that theophylline has a narrow toxicity-benefit range. Too little is of no use. Too much can cause headaches, jitteriness, stomach upset, and seizures. The buffer between the good and bad effects is narrow, and people vary in how they absorb the drug. So prescribing theophylline is an art.

Nevertheless the drug works. Certain people respond particularly well. And it can be helpful when used properly.

G. Sansone has come to rescue theophylline from oblivion where it seemed headed. The doctor studied theophylline's anti-inflammatory potential. These days this is quite important. Current treatment emphasizes how crucial it is to reduce inflammation in the lungs. By showing that theophylline could block the inflammation due to nitrous oxide in certain asthmatic patients, Dr. Sansone may have given theophylline a new life. If others confirm his findings that theophylline is anti-inflammatory and can take the place of cortisone-steroid-type drugs in certain patients, this will be good news because we like to avoid cortisone-steroids when we can.

Helpful hint 1: Drugs may fall out of favor and still be useful. The trick is to learn what the problems are and tailor treatment accordingly. As some people say, you don't need to throw the baby out with the bath water.

Helpful hint 2: Some people feel it is easier to throw the baby out with the bath water than to take the trouble to figure out how to keep the baby and still get rid of the dirty bath water.

Theophylline Can Cause Emotional Problems In Children

Dr. Clifton Furukawa studied theophylline and found that in addition to overt side effects like nausea, headaches, jitteriness, and an abnormal heartbeat, theophylline can also be responsible for subtle behavioral and learning problems in children. If you notice that your child's behavior changes, he has sleeping difficulty, or he develops a learning disability, *or* if teachers notice such changes *and* if the child is using theophylline, consult your child's doctor. Most behavioral and learning disorders are *not* due to theophylline, but it is worth considering.

Helpful hint 1: If you give medication to a child and notice a change in the way the child feels, acts or behaves, consult your doctor to see if the change is possibly due to the medication.

Tests For Theophylline Drug Level And Why The Tests Are Frequently Unnecessary

When treating asthma with theophylline, most allergists aim to keep the blood level between ten and fifteen micrograms. To measure the level, allergists used to have to send a blood sample to an outside laboratory.

Now there are tests that enable your doctors to perform the measurement in their office. This makes it easier to keep track of the efficacy of your treatment. In some offices the blood level is measured at every visit to determine if the dose needs to be changed.

Dr. Charles Reed examined the practice of frequent testing. He concluded it is unnecessary to test everyone's theophylline *routinely*. Several studies have shown that low to moderate doses (even below ten micrograms) are sufficient to control asthma in most people. So there is no need to put every person who takes theophylline on a high dose, subject them to possible side effects, and require them to undergo constant monitoring with blood tests.

Dr. Reed, who works at the Mayo Clinic, went so far as to say that only the *severest* cases of asthma must be given high doses of theophylline that are close to toxic levels and which require frequent monitoring.

Helpful hint 1: If you take theophylline and feel side effects, ask your doctor to test you to determine whether you are taking too much.

Helpful hint 2: Theophylline blood levels don't have to be done routinely. The major exception is when you must be hospitalized for a severe attack and your doctor feels high doses might help break the attack.

Helpful hint 3 There are certain drugs and several illnesses that can raise or lower the theophylline level. This can create toxic effects from too much or render theophylline ineffective from too little a dose.

Decrease Theophylline Level	Raise Theophylline Level
1. Young children	1. Tagamet
2. Smoking	2. Liver disease
3. High protein diet	3. Erythromycin
4. Phenobarbital	4. Viral infection
5. Phenytoin	5. Heart failure
	6. Pneumonia

Helpful hint 4: It is not wrong for your doctors to *routinely* test for theophylline, but do not be overly impressed that routine tests indicate you are receiving advanced medical treatment. In most cases, routine testing is not necessary.

Breaking Asthma Tablets To Obtain Half-Doses Can Be Dangerous

Doctors generally calculate the dose of asthma medication based on your body size and the severity of your symptoms, which, as you probably know from your own experience, depends on the degree of your exposure, the season of the year, whether you have a secondary infection, and many other factors. Thus, for a variety of reasons your doctor may tell you to break your allergy tablets in half so you can take a half, a whole, or one-and-a-half pills.

Dr. Cheryl Lutz discovered that breaking the 100 mg size of a pill called Theo-Dur may cause problems even though the tablet is scored, which indicates that it was designed to be broken in half.

Dr. Lutz measured the blood levels of theophylline, which is the active ingredient in Theo-Dur, and found that the halves produced unequal relief compared to the whole. In some cases one half of the tablet was absorbed faster than the other half. Thus the time to reach maximum blood level varied. This resulted in less predictable control of symptoms and greater tendency to experience side effects.

Helpful hint 1: If you notice an unusual response when you use a half-tablet or half-capsule of medication, consult your doctor.

Latest and Greatest High-Tech Asthma Drug

Drug companies are always looking for new medications. They design a drug based on an idea, conduct animal studies, move to human studies, and finally mass market the product. Currently they are working on several promising anti-asthma drugs which have been shown to counteract one or another of the chemical mediators that cause asthma.

As you read in an earlier chapter, allergic diseases such as asthma occur when allergens enter your body, attach to IgE antibody, and cause certain of your cells to secrete chemical mediators. You could say that allergens cause your body to use your own chemicals against you.

The idea of your body making the chemicals that harm you may sound bizarre, but this is how many diseases occur. For example, your thyroid gland can excrete excess thryoid hormone and cause hyperthyroidism. The pancreas can manufacture too much insulin and cause hypoglycemia. The brain can fire off unnecessary electrical impulses and cause epilepsy. In these cases your body is trying to self-destruct.

Examples of bodily-produced chemicals that make asthma are histamine, 5-lipoxygenase, adhesion molecules, and leukotrienes, to name just a few. We have an antidote for histamine, and thanks to gene research and genetic engineering doctors are making anti-everything-else these days, too.

Dr. Sally Wenzel has studied the new "anti-mediator" drugs. She found that they help, but they aren't yet as effective as the current bronchodilators and steroids. Some names you may hear are Zileuton, Rolipram, Siguazodan, Benafentrin, and Zaprinast.

Although these drugs haven't been the miracle we've been hoping for, hopefully the miracle will come along.

In any case, get ready for more drugs with strange names that counteract chemicals in your body that have even stranger names.

In the meantime, take the drugs that your doctor gives you and follow your doctor's instructions. Be a good patient. Your doctor will sleep better at night, and so will you.

Helpful hint 1: Don't wait for modern science to find a miracle cure for asthma and allergy. Take your old-fashioned, traditional medicine and be well. When something *really* useful comes along, your doctor will let you know and you can switch to the new drug.

Serious Deficiencies That Have Been Noted In The Treatment Of Asthma

Dr. Charles Reed, who has already been quoted several times in this book, discovered facts about the treatment of asthma that will astound you.

Doctors have more effective drugs for the treatment of asthma and greater numbers of them than at any time in history. We have deeper understanding of the mechanisms by which allergy produces asthma symptoms. Anyone with common sense would predict that it is easier to control asthma and we are getting better results. But the facts show the opposite!

In the six years from 1977 to 1983, the cost of medicine purchased for asthma shot up two and one half times from 144 million dollars to 362 million dollars (corrected for inflation), and it is still rising. Despite the increased use of anti-asthma drugs, the number of patients who had to be admitted to hospitals for asthma doubled from ten to twenty admissions per 10,000 people. How can a country spend twice as much money on advanced drugs and yet have results that are twice as bad?

Scientists theorized that the increased number of hospital admissions had to be due to an increased number of people getting asthma. With bad air, chemical pollution, unhealthy diets, smoking, and so forth this explanation made a lot of sense until scientific studies showed that the number of asthmatics had not changed.

Next, scientists wondered if the problem was peculiar to the United States where it could be blamed on smog or acid rain. But studies showed that other countries had a high death rate, too.

How Can We Be Spending More to Achieve Less?

Dr. Reed didn't know the answer to the above question. Neither do I. But it is interesting to speculate.

One possibility is that doctors rely too much on drugs and therefore ignore the fundamentals of proper allergy treatment which is educating you about avoiding allergens and teaching you how to use your medication.

Each new drug gets rave reviews, and I can understand why it is easy to believe that all you need to do is take a pill and the pill will do the work. This is nowhere near the truth. Not even close. What's needed is a full discussion and understanding of when, why, how, and where a person's allergy problems occur. Then the *patient* needs to study how to keep away from allergens and practice starting and stopping his medication until he is a professional asthma patient.

Talking to Patients Has Gone the Way of the Dinosaur

We, both you and we doctors, cannot afford to rely on high-tech tests and "new and powerful" drugs. We need to restore our faith in old-fashioned treatments like getting rid of the cat and stopping cigarette smoking. This isn't easy. Our busy lifestyles and the pressures of managed care conspire against us. It is easier and faster for a busy doctor to give you a drug than to try to convince you to stop smoking or get rid of your cat. Likewise, it probably easier for you to accept a drug than listen to a lecture about stopping smoking or getting rid of your cat.

If asthma statistics were improving, these considerations might not matter. But the statistics are not improving. They are getting worse! I may be considered old-fashioned for saying this, but I believe that returning to the fundamentals of allergy treatment, which means that we doctors take the time to listen to your story, do a thorough evaluation, explain how to use medication, and discuss proper avoidance, can get us back on the path to proper allergy treatment.

There is a trend toward using video films and slide shows in medical offices. I'm afraid this is worsening the situation. Busy doctors are thinking, "I know I can't sit down and talk to each patient as long as I should, so I'll show them a video tape. My patients can watch the video and get the same information I would give them. This will fulfill my obligation."

Although these offices might mean well, they overlook the fact that there is no substitute for a face to face explanation. When I sit face-to-face with a patient, I can tell from his expressions what information he has grasped and what I must repeat in greater detail. I can also tailor what he must do to his particular problem instead of giving the same *generic* instructions to everyone. Although videos and slides are better than nothing, they aren't as effective as having your own, *personal* trainer.

I use the term trainer because an asthmatic needs training. You need to learn what to do, when to do it, how to do it, and when to stop. In fact, stopping medication is often as important as knowing when to start. On the other side of the coin, *you*, the patient, need to listen, take notes, and be willing to follow instructions.

I'm sorry but we have no miracle cures. Until we find a miracle, taking care of asthma will be hard work. And you are the one who must do the work. So you must *demand* that your doctors talk to you and tell you how long it takes to judge whether a particular drug is working, how to use your drugs, what are the side effects, and how to figure out whether you can reduce the dose or even stop.

Many treatments fail not because they are bad but because they are not used properly. For example, in the chapter on nasal sprays you read that you must use each spray a particular way, the way it was designed, or there is no point using it at all.

Another explanation for our poor results in treating asthma and preventing asthma deaths is that many types of health care professional treat allergy (see, Will The Real Allergist Please Stand Up?). I've been told it is a matter of opinion what type of doctor is best qualified to treat allergic asthma, but it seems to me that an allergist who has spent several extra years studying and specializing is a better bet.

Whatever the actual reason for the poor statistics in asthma care, doctors must consider mundane possibilities, like talking to you more, not focusing exclusively on expensive research, and not hoping that the latest high-tech drug will do the job by itself. By the same token, you must be willing to cooperate with your doctors instead of expecting a miracle.

Helpful hint 1: Considering the advances that have been made in the field of allergy and allergic asthma, it is hard to understand why people throughout the world are having more asthma than they used to.

Helpful hint 2: If you have asthma, you are more likely to be treated successfully if you consult a doctor who is trained to take care of your illness.

Helpful hint 3: A new high-tech drug is not necessarily a better drug.

12

Cortisone-Steroids for Allergic Disease

From the day I began my allergy training over twenty-five years ago, (I shudder to think how long that is) I've listened to certain professors recommend that we treat all allergy problems with cortisone-steroids. After learning about allergy, I can understand why they would say this. This family of drugs is almost guaranteed to alleviate symptoms.

On the other hand cortisone-steroids have certain long-term permanent side effects. So there was always a group of physicians who urged caution in using these drugs. Well, all this changed when pharmaceutical companies developed new ways of using cortisone-steroids such as inhalers and new types of cortisone that were more potent and required less frequent dosing. In fact the small but vocal chorus in favor of cortisone has grown to a symphony. With managed care insurance companies urging Primary Care Doctors to treat diseases that used to go to a specialist, the symphony has reached a crescendo that is deafening. This movement has come to the point where many people seem to have forgotten or are ignoring well-known and dangerous facts about cortisone-steroids.

I must warn you in advance that parts of this chapter are the opposite of what you will hear from the National

Institutes of Health, many respected professors, and some of my colleagues. Nevertheless I cannot give up my healthy respect for the bad things cortisone-steroids do just because it is an easy way out to treat allergy.

Everything in life has its advantages and disadvantages, and cortisone-steroids are no exception. It is only fair that you hear *both* sides of the cortisone-steroid story. Then you can discuss this with your doctors and make your own *informed* decision.

The Best Way To Take Cortisone (Steroids)

Cortisone is one of those drugs that could be called a miracle. It is used for cancer, allergy, arthritis, and brain surgery, to name just a handful of the hundreds of diseases for which it is frequently prescribed.

One of the paradoxes of cortisone is that your own body makes it. Each night your body measures the amount of cortisone circulating in your bloodstream and makes enough for your next day's needs.

However, your body can't tell the difference between cortisone that comes from a pill and cortisone that it has made itself. So if you take cortisone medication, the adrenal gland, which is the tissue that makes cortisone-steroids, figures it doesn't have to make any. With disuse, the gland shrinks and atrophies just like your muscles shrink and become flabby when they are not used. If you develop a severe infection, need surgery, or suffer stress in which your body needs cortisone-type hormones, your adrenal gland, having been suppressed, isn't ready to produce. Atrophied muscles can take months to recover their full strength. Your adrenal gland can take up to a year.

Another danger from taking cortisone is the direct effect it has on tissues. This can lead to permanent damage such as cataracts in the eyes, softening of bones, possible fractures, delayed growth in children, and thinning of the skin. It produces short-term effects such as weight gain, ulcer, and psychological changes, too, but these effects are usually reversible.

Thus, due to the long-term permanent side effects, it is best to avoid cortisone-steroids. However, standard allergy treatments don't always help. So allergists often turn to cortisone-steroids. In many cases, the good effects outweigh the bad.

If you reach the point where your symptoms are bad and nothing is working, your doctor may prescribe cortisone-steroids. Begin with the smallest amount and work up. There is no point in taking more of this drug than you need. These are the five steps to sensible steroid use.

Most desirable method to take cortisone

This first step is tongue in cheek. The best way to take cortisone-steroid-type drugs is *not* to take them at all. The long-lasting, permanent side effects such as cataracts, softening of bones, delayed growth in children, and thinning of the skin are irreversible. The short-acting effects, the ones that subside from a few weeks to a few months after discontinuing the drug, are increased susceptibility to infection, weight gain, psychological changes, diabetes, and high blood pressure, to name just a few of the problems that can develop.

Second best way

Assuming you need cortisone, begin with a brief burst (like one or two weeks of Prednisone, Prednisolone, or Medrol) or a single intramuscular shot (Depo-Medrol). When used once a year, your body generallly won't absorb enough cortisone-steroid to produce long-term effects, although the short-term effects could still occur. However, if brief bursts or single, steroid shots are repeated frequently, they can quickly put you in one of the categories described below, even if they weren't intended to.

Third best way

The third step to avoid long-term side effects (although this may not avoid the short-term effects) is to use cortisone-steroid every other day. On the day you don't use cortisone your adrenal gland has an opportunity to recover.

When taking cortisone every other day, it is best to take the whole day's dose in the morning since this further reduces adrenal suppression. However, several studies have shown that taking cortisone-steroid in the afternoon produces the best effect so you may find yourself in a dilemma-whether to minimize the side effects by taking it in the morning or maximize the benefical effect by taking it in the afternoon. (Whoever said life would be simple?)

Fourth best way

The fourth way is to *inhale* cortisone. This puts the medication right in your lungs and nose. The *theory* is that cortisone-steroid will then only affect the local area where it is needed. Distant organs such as bones, muscles, and eyes wouldn't be affected.

Unfortunately, despite what certain manufacturers claim, cortisone is absorbed from skin surfaces. The more your skin is inflamed and irritated, the more you absorb. When you apply cortisone ointment to your outer skin, from fifteen to thirty percent can be absorbed. When you apply it to the skin of your eyes, nose, or lungs, an even greater proportion can be absorbed because the skin in these areas is so thin. If your membranes are inflamed, as in the case of allergy, even more can be absorbed. Thus, application directly where it's needed on the skin surfaces doesn't guarantee protection from *internal* cortisone side effects. Application to the skin is simply the equivalent of ingesting a small dose every day.

Dr. John Toogood measured the blood level of cortisone-steroid after using inhalers and found enough drug in the bloodstream to cause weakening of the bones (osteoporosis). Dr. H. Bisgaard detected adrenal suppression. These doctors proved that the cortisone in cortisone-steroid nasal sprays is absorbed and can cause long-term side effects.

Below is a partial list of topical cortisones. A complete list can be found in the *Physician's Desk Reference*, which you can probably find in your local library.

Eye cortisone
   Decadron Ophthalmic
   Inflamase

Nasal cortisone
   Beconase
   Decadron Turbinaire
   Flonase
   Nasacort
   Nasarel
   Rhinocort
   Vancenase
   Most "allergy shots" which are injected into the nose

Lung cortisone
   Aerobid
   Azmacort
   Beclovent
   Budesonide
   Dexacort
   Flovent
   Fluocortin Butyl
   Fluticasone
   Pulmicort
   Vanceril

Fifth best way

The fifth step is *daily* cortisone. At this point nothing has worked. You and your doctors' backs are against the wall.

Your doctor can start with a low dose and switch you to a high dose, if necessary. Neither of these are good choices. But when you have no choice, you have no choice. If you must use daily cortisone, you may have to take calcium and in some cases a hormone to prevent weakening of your bones.

Summary

After reading that there are five ways doctors prescribe cortisone, you can well imagine how easy it is for a patient to become confused. One time he may be told to take cortisone spray. Then he may be told to take pills every day, every other day, or in brief bursts.

As a person progresses from one level to another, the specific regimen may seem arbitrary and mysterious. But allergists have a logical reason based on maximizing the good effect and minimizing the bad.

Your goal should be to avoid cortisone. If you aren't successful, begin with bursts, move to every other day, and finally begin daily doses.

Just keep in mind that you and your doctor should do whatever you can to head in the direction of *not* using cortisone.

Helpful hint 1: Cortisone pills, shots, and sprays aren't the best thing for your body. Cortisone stops your adrenal gland from functioning and can cause other serious side effects.

Helpful hint 2: When you must use cortisone, there are techniques and regimens to minimize the side effects. We pray that researchers will discover other methods of taking care of allergies so that no one will have to take cortisone in the future.

Helpful hint 3: When you stop using cortisone-steroid, doctors often ask you to taper the dose gradually instead of abruptly. The reason is that in the normal situation, the adrenal gland must be able to make extra cortisone-steroid for medical emergencies like severe infections, surgery, or stress. In the situation where you have taken cortisone for a prolonged period, the adrenal gland is too weak to pump out extra hormone. So during the crossover period while the adrenal gland regains its strength, the trick is to *gradually* decrease the oral steroid while the body *gradually* increases its intrinsic steroid. Thus, you always have enough steroid for your needs.

Helpful hint 4: Despite the problems I've described, cortisone-steroids are extremely helpful. I wouldn't give them up for anything. It's comforting to know that a high enough dose can relieve almost any allergy problem. In a crisis, this can save your life.

Helpful hint 5: Cortisone is the "no-brain" treatment for allergy. If you don't care what's causing your problem, what side effects you might experience, or what's really underlying your allergy symptoms, use cortisone.

Best Time to Take Your Steroids

Since oral steroids can take a half day to become effective and inhaled steroids can take up to a week, you'd think the exact time you take this type of medicine would be unimportant. Wrong! Drs. Pincus and Gagnon showed you get the best results if you take cortisone-steroid at 3PM.

Previously, doctors had determined that you reduce the chance of serious side effects if you take cortisone-steroid type drugs between 6AM and 8AM.

So, doctors have proven that you can't just worry about remembering to take your medicine. You also need to choose between the best results and the least side effects.

Helpful hint 1: Sometimes medical studies prove you are damned if you do and damned if you don't.

13

Allergy Injections

The phrase "allergy injection" customarily refers to an injection of allergenic proteins that are derived from grasses, trees, weeds, dust, mold, and animal dander. Injecting these allergens builds *permanent* immunity in the same way that injecting viral agents like measles, mumps, and polio builds permanent immunity against infectious organisms.

Compare this to the kind of "allergy injection" in which a doctor gives you an injection of a medication for *temporary* relief.

To find out whether your doctor intends to give you the short-term, temporary or long-term, permanent type of injection, you need to ask him.

Since immunizing injections contain the substances that cause your symptoms, allergists build the dose gradually. A typical series can take twenty to twenty-five visits to reach what's called maintenance level. The injections continue, usually once a month, for three to five years. At completion, most people have permanent immunity.

Short-term injections simply give you temporary relief which lasts from a few hours to a week depending on the particular drug that's prescribed.

The first section of this chapter is an overview of both the drug- and allergen-containing injections. The remaining sections deal exclusively with the allergen-containing, immunizing injections. You will read about a polymerized serum that doctors had hoped would allow patients to achieve life-time immunity with fifteen shots, why it is important for you to stay on an immunizing-injection program faithfully, how to prevent allergy serum from deteriorating, why you need a specialist to figure out how to combine allergens in an allergy extract, how to prevent injections from failing, how doctors are experimenting with oral and sublingual drops as a substitute for allergy injections, how often you should be retested to decide whether you can stop allergy injections, the results of using injections for food allergy, and finally the latest, high-tech type of injection that was developed using advanced molecular biology.

The One Shot Cure For Allergies

Every so often a patient asks if I will give them one shot that will cure their allergies. Usually they've heard about such an injection from a relative or a friend.

There are many kinds of injections for allergy. Each one is used for a different purpose. Several are "one shot". Several are not. Below is a complete list of allergy injections. If you hear about "one shot", refer to the list and figure out whether it is the kind that would be appropriate for you.

There are nine categories of injections. Categories five and six are the only ones that contain natural substances which boost your immunity to counteract excessive levels of IgE antibody. Since excess IgE is the underlying cause of allergy, these two types of shots are the only ones capable of producing permanent immunity. The remaining seven types are merely drugs which relieve symptoms *on a temporary basis.*

1. Epinephrine (adrenalin)

Epinephrine is a drug that is used to treat acute attacks of asthma, outbreaks of hives, and sudden anaphylaxis. Anaphylaxis is the most feared of allergic reactions because it begins with lightning speed and can end up in death.

Epinephrine injections last about fifteen to twenty minutes. They usually bring a reaction under control within five to ten minutes so there is an extra ten-minute safety valve. When epinephrine wears off, a reaction can sometimes come back so occasionally a doctor needs to give a second injection. Epinephrine is an old, old remedy and is the first-line drug for allergic emergencies.

If you are susceptible to sudden, severe, life-threatening allergic reactions, ask your doctor to prescribe an epinephrine syringe. After all, your doctor isn't with you twenty-four hours a day, and you can't depend on being close to an emergency room if a severe allergic reaction hits. Two common epinephrines are Ana-kit and Epi-pen. Ana-kit has two doses per syringe. Epi-pen has one dose. With Ana-kit you inject yourself. With Epi-pen you push a button that activates a spring that pushes the needle.

2. Sus-Phrine

Sus-Phrine contains epinephrine in a form that lasts eight to twelve hours. Your doctor will use this so he doesn't have to give you plain epinephrine every twenty minutes in cases where the rection is expected to be prolonged. and is prescribed for acute asthma and hives. Like epinephrine it has been available for a long time.

3. Albuterol

Albuterol is a *modified* epinephrine. It lasts about thirty to sixty minutes. Allergists use it for acute attacks of asthma and hives just like we use epinephrine for asthma and hives.

Dr. Sheldon Spector found that albuterol was an improvement over epinephrine in certain patients. For others it was not.

Strictly speaking, albuterol isn't new. It's been available for many years in tablets, liquids, and inhalers. Using it as an injection is a new technique.

4. Terbutaline

Terbutaline is another epinephrine-like drug. In a few people it causes less stimulation of the heart and less jitteriness than epinephrine.

5. Allergy Immunizing Injections

Allergy immunizing injections contain no drugs. Instead, they contain natural substances like grasses, weeds, trees, dust, mold, and animal dander. Allergists increase the dose each week to force your body to make immunity.

Generally you need about twenty injections to reach a dose where you take an injection once a month. After three years, you can usually stop. By then most patients have a kind of permanent immunity (see the section on Three Treatments of Allergy for details).

Immunizing injections have been used for several decades with great safety in all ages and even during pregnancy. Their chief advantage is they attack your underlying problem and contain no drugs that could produce unwanted or deleterious side effects. The price you pay for trying to achieve a cure is that this treatment is definitely not "one shot".

6. Peptides

Peptides are small fragments of a parent protein. Doctors make them using high-tech, modern, gene technology. They are the core of the molecules that stimulate IgE and cause allergic reactions. The rest of the molecule just carries this core to where it can affect you and do the most damage.

Scientists have figured out how to tailor the molecule to leave out the part that causes allergic reactions but still leave enough of the molecule behind so that you will make immunity to the *overall* molecule. This allows us to inject high doses without causing symptoms. The higher the dose, the more antibodies you make. The more antibodies you make, the better you can fight off allergens and the better you will feel.

Dr. Philip Norman at Johns Hopkins Hospital found that peptide immunotherapy was promising. His patients tolerated the injections, their symptoms improved, and the dose he was able to give them was quite high. On the other hand, two of nineteen patients had generalized reactions and had to stop peptide therapy. So this new type of extract, while it sounded promising, caused reactions just like standard therapy can. Thus, peptides will have to be used just as cautiously as our traditional extracts.

Furthermore, doctors will have to show peptide therapy is more effective than traditional treatment, or else the effort, while exciting from a scientific point of view, will have no practical application. It might merely substitute an expensive, high-tech technique for our current highly effective, traditional technique .

Allervax is the name of the peptide therapy that's currently hot. Undoubtedly there will be others. Look for them over the next few years. Also look for information about safety. Making these peptides is relatively easy. Proving they are safe and effective takes time. It is too early to tell whether peptides might create a long term problem. Several allergists have been concerned that these peptides could combine with proteins in the body, create new molecules, and trigger a worse problem than the original one.

Additionally scientists must learn how to make Allervax-type products for *all* allergens. Otherwise you will be forced to take traditional therapy for non-Allervax allergens *in addition to* Allervax-type therapy. This would force you into two different treatment schedules when before Allervax came along you only had to deal with one kind of treatment.

7. Antihistamines
If you have an acute allergic reaction such as after eating a food, doctors often inject an antihistamine. The most common one is Benadryl (also called diphenhydramine). Antihistamine injections last about four to six hours and like all drugs merely provide temporary relief.

8. Cortison-steroid
Cortisone-steroid, which you've already read about, is a man-made steroid that duplicates a steroid hormone that the body produces on its own. When used as a medication cortisone-steroid suppresses inflammation in tissues throughout the body. We use it to alleviate arthritis, sports injuries, allergies, third degree burns, certain types of cancer, and other problems that are too numerous to mention.

There are a many brands of cortisone-steroid. They are sold in liquid, tablet, intravenous, ointment, inhalation, and intramuscular preparations.

Cortisone injections can persist in your body up to three weeks. This will almost always stop allergy symptoms. Cortisone won't build your immunity, but it sure feels good! If your allergy season is brief, this single shot will appear to have cured you. If your season lasts longer than three or four weeks, you may need several cortisone injections to carry you through. Of course next year your symptoms will return and force you to take more cortisone. People tend to forget this. Instead they just remember that cortisone stopped their symptoms and made them feel better.

Unfortunately cortisone can cause serious side effects like ulcer, weight gain, cataracts, softening of bones, and high blood pressure. These effects are dangerous. Unlike the short-term side effects of other allergy medication such as sleepinees, jitteriness, and nausea that can occur with antihistamines and bronchodilators, cortisone-steroid's side effects may not go away even after you stop using the drug.

I suppose you could call a cortisone-steroid injection an allergy shot. I prefer to call it an injection of a drug which can stop symptoms for a period of time. When cortisone wears off, you must take it again. Examples of brands of injectable cortisone are Aristocort, Celestone, Decadron, Depo-Medrol, Dexamethasone, Kenalog, and Solu-Cortef.

9. Nasal Cortisone Shot

Nasal cortisone injections don't differ from other cortisone injections. I listed them separately because of the myth that when cortisone is injected into your nose it cannot produce side effects. No matter where or how cortisone is given, this drug is eventually absorbed into your body. Even when applied to your skin, cortisone is absorbed and can produce serious cortisone side effects.

Dr. Ray Slavin reported that the United States Food and Drug Administration has considered banning nasal cortisone shots because several people lost their vision. Losing your vision is a high price to pay to stop sneezing.

There are different brand names of cortisone-steroid that disguise the fact that it is a steroid. So you may not know that you are getting a steroid unless you ask. The appendix lists some of the brands to help you figure this out. Nevertheless, if you hear someone got a nasal injection for their allergy symptoms, you can be fairly certain they got a cortisone-steroid.

I hope it's clear by now that cortisone, whether administered into your nose, muscle, or vein, is not a sure-fire, one-shot, quick cure. It can provide temporary relief for up to three weeks at a time. This may feel like a cure. The problem is those darn side effects.

Helpful hint 1: There is no "one-shot" cure for allergy.

Helpful hint 2: There are two types of injections for allergy. One type contains various drugs that relieve your symptoms for a finite length of time. The other type is immunizing injections which contain no medicine. Instead immunizing injections build your immunity to the substances such as dust, pets, and pollens that are responsible for your allergic reactions.

Helpful hint 3: Although you may not be told you are being given cortisone, a nasal injection that is said to be "one-shot for your allergies" strongly indicates you are getting cortisone.

New Type Of Allergy Injection Means Fewer Shots (Polymerized Extract)

Dr. Roy Patterson of Chicago spent many years attempting to improve allergy serum so that immunizing injections could be given less often and with greater safety.

For ragweed- and grass-allergic patients, Dr. Patterson developed a special serum called polymerized serum. Using this material, he gave twenty injections and produced permanent immunity in certain individuals.

Dr. Patterson accomplished this by altering molecules of ragweed and grass pollen. If you're not familiar with how allergy injections work, you'd have to understand the theory behind injection therapy in order to understand how Dr. Patterson succeeded with his special serum.

Ordinary allergy injections contain extracts of grasses, trees, weeds, dust, mold, and animal dander. These are the very substances to which you are allergic. There is no medication in them, no drugs of any kind.

Since you are allergic to the ingredients, allergists raise the dose a little at a time to prevent a reaction. After approximately twenty build-up injections, which are given once or twice a week, patients reach a point that is called maintenance level. From then on, the injections are given every three to four weeks to maintain the immunity. At the end of three years, allergists try to stop treatment since, by then, most patients have permanent immunity. If you are asked to take injections longer than three years without even attempting to stop, this probably means your doctors are using the low- instead of the high-dose method, although even at high doses *certain* patients cannot stop.

The secret of Dr. Patterson's success was in finding a way to separate the allergy-provoking ability of allergens from their immune-stimulating ability. This enabled him to give larger doses of serum per injection without fear of an allergic reaction. It is similar to the feat scientists achieved when they figured out how to suppress the infection-producing and increase the immune-stimulating property of polio, measles, and mumps viruses. Thus, when pediatricians vaccinate children, the children get better not worse, even though they are being injected with organisms that are ordinarily harmful.

With polymerized serum, Dr. Patterson was able to inject large amounts of pollen whose allergy-provoking potential had been blunted. Thus, each of his doses stimulated his patients to make huge quantities of antibodies without causing symptoms. Previously, allergists needed to administer several injections of standard serum to achieve the same immunity as one injection of Dr. Patterson's serum. With more immunity per injection, patients not only went longer between injections, they achieved better results, too.

There are several disadvantages to these new injections, however. Dr. Patterson has not made polymerized serum for dog, cat, or mold. Therefore, if you are allergic to dog, cat, or mold, you would have to take traditional injections too. This would actually *increase* the number of shots you'd need. Secondly, these substances haven't been used long enough to know if they are safe for prolonged periods of time. Traditional injections contain natural substances such as grasses, weeds, trees, and dog dander. These allergens enter your body whenever you breathe. And being natural, they are not inherently dangerous, unless you are allergic to them.

Polymerized serum is made with *altered* molecules, though. This makes them *unnatural*. Only time will tell whether they are completely harmless. Finally, not everyone who took polymerized injections was completely cured after twenty shots. Most of the patients Dr. Patterson treated had to continue the injections for three or four years just as do those who receive traditional allergy serum.

Helpful hint 1: Injections of polymerized serum are not really new. Dr. Roy Patterson and other groups of doctors have been studying them for almost twenty years.

Helpful hint 2: There are several researchers who polymerize serum by a different technique from Dr. Patterson's. At the present time, no one is certain whose method is best.

Helpful hint 3: Those of you who are allergic to dust, pets, mold, and feathers would need injections of *traditional* serum for dust, pets, mold, and feathers *in addition* to polymerized serum for ragweed and grasses. Instead of reducing your visits and shots, this would actually increase the number of injections you would need.

Helpful hint 4: Although there may be less risk of systemic reactions with polymerized sera, systemic reactions still occur. In the hands of people who have taken specialized allergy training, the systemic reaction rate using traditional sera is 0.45 percent. The statistics which have been published from Dr. Patterson's group using polymerized sera show a rate of 0.35 percent. Thus, although polymerized serum reduces the reaction rate, the reduction is only a slight improvement on what is already a well-controlled problem.

Helpful hint 5: No one knows the long term effects of injecting serum, such as polymerized serum, which contains altered proteins. Tests of immune function have shown no adverse effects from traditional extracts which contain natural proteins. But polymerized extract has not been used by many people and must now enter the "consumer is guinea pig" stage. Doctors do not know for sure where this will lead.

Helpful hint 6: As with any new drug, treatment, or procedure there are pros and cons. Usually in such situations, the ultimate answer is that a certain segment of patients can be treated with polymerized serum successfully while others will need traditional serum. Always remember that a treatment that is helpful for *select* individuals is not necessarily helpful for *all* individuals.

New Polymerized Serum May Not Be Better Than Traditional Serum

Working in France, Dr. Jean Bousquet treated patients with a special polymerized serum and discovered that doses of 5,000 units of polymerized allergen extracts achieve the same immunity as with 80,000 polymerized units. Interestingly, 5,000 units is the dose used by allergists who use traditional serum and adhere to the high dose method of treatment.

So if Dr. Bousquet's findings are confirmed, this means there is nothing to be gained by giving 80,000 units. You might as well stick to the traditional extract and traditional dosing of 5,000 units. Of course, if you are not being treated with high doses of traditional allergy extract, you would do better with the polymerized-type extracts.

Helpful hint 1: Although polymerized allergy serum seemed to be a great advance, preliminary information from Dr. Jean Bousquet's laboratory shows that super-high doses of polymerized serum produce no better results than the *recommended* dose of traditional serum.

Helpful hint 2: Those medical offices which routinely use low-dose injections ought to reconsider and begin reserving low doses only for those patients who cannot tolerate the recommended high doses.

How Pollen Can Bother You After The Pollen Season Ends

At the end of your pollen season, you and your allergist have every reason to expect your symptoms to diminish as the pollen count drops. Unfortunately, your expectations are not always fulfilled. Several doctors in Minnesota found out why from studying patients who are allergic to red oak trees.

After the red oak season ended, the doctors discovered significant amounts of red oak pollen on the ground. When the wind blew, this pollen became airborne and triggered symptoms in oak-allergic patients. Since this can happen with other pollens as well, you can see why you may feel ill after your season ends and why you may need to continue your treatment longer than you might have anticipated.

Helpful hint 1: Certain of you who have pollen allergies may have to continue allergy immunizing injections *and allergy medication* beyond your traditional pollinating season due to pollen that has blown to the ground during the active pollenating season and *recirculates* after the season is supposed to have ended.

Discovery That Allergy Serum Loses Potency Quickly

Allergy serum loses its strength when it is exposed to warm temperatures. This is called *thermal* decay. To prevent this from happening, allergists store your serum in a refrigerator. Even at refrigerator temperatures, though, your serum can lose its potency with the passage of time due to *spontaneous* decay.

Dr. Harold Nelson studied the decay phenomenon and found that over the course of several months bottles of sera are removed from the refrigerator many times in order to prepare injections for each appointment. Thus, each bottle of serum undergoes many days of warming and can become unacceptably weak.

This is a serious problem because the weaker the serum the less immunity it will stimulate and the less effective are allergy shots.

The most commonly used sera are the aqueous or watery ones, even though these are subject to the fastest deterioration. The slowest to lose strength are glycerin- and albumin-based. Although doctors have known that aqueous are the most susceptible to decay, many medical offices ignore this and continue to use the aqueous solution because the glycerinated kind can sting you for a moment.

My teachers, Drs. William Deamer and Lee Frick, insisted that glycerin be used because this kind of serum retains its potency best. Furthermore, despite the *theoretical* possibility of stinging, very few patients actually have problems. Thus, it does not make sense to use weaker and less effective solutions when the vast majority of people tolerate the strong and active material.

In addition to sera that deteriorate quickly, there is a serum that is actually weak from the start. This is the situation with a serum called Allpyral. Allpyral is made by a unique process. Many years ago Dr. Larry Lichtenstein at

Johns Hopkins Medical School showed that this process weakens the ingredients so that they don't stimulate immunity as strongly as the standard extracts that most companies make.

However, Allpyral is of inestimable help for super-sensitive patients who cannot tolerate standard allergy extracts. However, since the majority of patients aren't super-sensitive, doctors who prescribe Allpyral *exclusively* are treating all their patients with less than the full immunizing doses which their patients might be capable of tolerating.

Helpful hint 1: It's better to have burning and stinging for a few minutes than to take injections that don't burn or sting but are so weak they don't do much good.

Helpful hint 2: The stronger the serum injected, the more immunity you make. The more immunity you make, the longer you can go between injections and the fewer doctor visits you'll need.

Helpful hint 3: You can tell your doctor that you would prefer strong serum and you are willing to put up with a little burning in order to take advantage of the benefits of strong allergy serum. Besides, despite the talk of burning and stinging, most people tolerate strong injections without difficulty.

Generic Allergy Extract and Dust Mite Can Ruin Your Chance For Successful Immunization

The immune system can respond to several allergens in the same injection just as infants can respond to two or three vaccinations in the same syringe. So to save you from needing ten or more injections for each and every allergen, allergists usually put a *mixture* of allergens in their allergy extracts. In this way they can immunize you to several substances at the same time.

However, making mixtures requires a certain expertise. One problem is the practice of making *generic* mixtures, Due to a large volume of patients, certain medical offices and clinics prescribe generic mixtures. Thus, everyone who is allergic to trees gets the tree mixture, to weeds they get the weed mixture, and so forth. This is easier than making and storing special bottles for each patient. But generic mixtures assume that everyone is sensitive to the identical substances to the same degree. As you probably know, each person's allergies are *different*. Despite this, many people obtain satisfactory relief from generic mixtures.

Dr. S. Kagan discovered another problem. Certain enzymes found in dust mite attack and weaken other allergens such as grasses, trees, and weeds. If dust mite is in your serum this would weaken the other ingredients and reduce the level of immunity your body can attain.

There are several ways to avoid these problems: ask for personalized mixtures, keep serum cold, use glycerin extract, and maintain separate bottles for dust mite injections.

Helpful hint 1: Mixing allergens may seem simple. But, like many aspects of allergy, there are many considerations such as the number of ingredients, their relative strength, and the type of fluid that's used.

New Reason Found For Injection Failure In Ragweed Allergy

Ragweed is one of the most bothersome and allergenic plants in the United States. Its pollen affects people wherever it is found. Fortunately for us on the West Coast, we have very little ragweed. East of the Rocky Mountains, though, ragweed is a major problem.

Ragweed produces so much pollen that the number of grains can be easily counted. So during ragweed season, radio stations in the East and Midwest report the pollen count beginning from the middle of August until early October. In case you aren't already miserable with ragweed symptoms, these reports remind you how sick you should be.

Interestingly many of the reports count every grain as a ragweed grain even though some of the pollens come from other plants. The theory behind this obvious mistake is that ragweed makes up ninety percent of Fall pollen so it doesn't matter what the other ten percent is and therefore it is not worth the extra effort to identify and count each and every species separately.

Well, I can tell you, now, that Dr. John Santilli, found that it does make a difference what those other pollens are. Dr. Santilli noticed that some of his ragweed-sensitive patients did not feel better after taking ragweed-allergy injections. Upon investigation, he discovered that these patients were allergic to molds which are found in high concentration at the same time of year ragweed is in the air. By neglecting mold and excluding it from these patients' serums, the patients' treatment was incomplete.

Only when your doctors search for *all* possibilities and treat you for *all* your sensitivities will you obtain optimum relief.

Helpful hint 1: Even if you have a classic history for a particular allergy such as fall ragweed allergy, your doctors should consider *all* possibilities before they make a final decision on how to treat you.

Helpful hint 2: If you have ragweed allergy and aren't obtaining satisfactory relief, ask your doctor to reevaluate you. You may be one of those who has mold allergy, too.

Oral Drops Might Replace Allergy Injections

Dr. Ebbe Taudorf, who does research in Denmark, tried to immunize patients by a unique method. His idea was to dissolve pollen in a special solution and administer this *orally* in gradually increasing quantities to allergic individuals and thus immunize them. This would save them from a course of allergy injections. Other physicians had tried a similar approach but had had no success.

In Dr. Taudorf's hands, oral weed treatment gave patients partial immunity against allergic reactions to weeds. Unfortunately, grass treatment did not give immunity. Another disappointment was that the oral drops helped eye symptoms but did not help nasal symptoms.

Furthermore, the drops were not innocuous. Many patients suffered from diarrhea and abdominal pain due to gastrointestinal allergic reactions to the ingested allergens.

Dr. Taudorf plans to experiment with different doses of drops and even with tablets to see if he can increase the beneficial effect and minimize the undesirable effects. So far, though, he doesn't have the final answer.

Dr. Alain de Weck from Switzerland, Dr. H. Morrow Brown from England, and Dr. G. W. Canonica from The University of Genoa in Italy wrote about another oral immunizing technique. These doctors have found that *sublingual* drops, where you hold the drops under your tongue until they are absorbed, showed promising results for allergy to dust mite, grass pollen, cat, and birch tree. What's best is that this can be done at home. No more allergy visits!

So far adverse reactions to sublingual drops are few and far between. However, sublingual drops have been used in only a few patients. Until there is greater experience and wider knowledge of how, when, and what dose works, let others do the testing.

Helpful hint 1: Physicians are searching for a reliable technique to replace allergy injections. So far, they haven't figured out a foolproof replacement.

Helpful hint 2: If you suffer from allergy to airborne pollens and are waiting for an easy cure so you don't have to start allergy injections, you should probably go ahead with injections now instead of waiting for a medical breakthrough that may never come to pass.

How Often To Repeat The Skin Tests and Can Retesting Tell You When To Stop Shots

Should your skin tests be performed once in a lifetime or once a year? Is it useful to do them at the end of a series of allergy injections or in the middle?

Dr. T. Coleman studied these questions. From his investigations, he concluded that you need skin tests to diagnose your allergic problem. But you don't need to repeat the tests on a regular basis.

Your allergies do not vary from day to day, week to week, month to month, or even from year to year. Over several years your sensitivities might change, but, generally speaking, the changes would be minimal.

Additionally, Dr. Coleman's studies confirmed what allergists had known for many years: The results of scratch tests won't determine when you are ready to stop allergy injections.

You would think that retesting would help your doctors decide the appropriate time to stop injections. After all, if you have completed several years of injections, it is only reasonable to suppose that you could compare your initial tests to tests after being on shots and figure out if you have built your immunity to the point where you can discontinue your shots.

Unfortunately, the body doesn't work that way. Studies always show that you are *less sensitive* to allergens after injections. This indicates that your immunity has *increased* as a result of the injections. However, this does not indicate that you can stop your shots. It doesn't indicate you need to continue them, either.

To everyone's dismay, Dr. Coleman proved this point with a clever experiment. He treated patients, stopped their shots, observed how they felt off shots, and divided them into two groups based on whether they were able to stop shots with or without a relapse. Then he compared test results.

Upon reviewing the medical records and comparing pre- and post-shot test results, Dr. Coleman could not find a way to predict who would be successful stopping shots. Neither blood nor skin tests nor physical examination told him the answer. He concluded there was only one way to find out whether a patient could stop injections without a relapse. The patient had to stop the injections and see what their body would do.

The reason allergy tests aren't useful at predicting the outcome is that they indicate your level of immunity *at the time the tests are performed*. If you wish to use a test that can determine whether you will be successful stopping shots, you will need a test that tells you what your immunity level will be *after* you stop the shots. Will it stay high or drop off? Will it drop slowly or quickly? As you are aware, you need a crystal ball to predict anything, *including* what will happen if you stop allergy injections. At the present time, no one is making good crystal balls.

Are there situations where it is appropriate to be retested? Yes. If you develop a sudden change in your symptoms, if many years (five to ten) have elapsed since your initial tests were performed, or if you move to an area which has *significantly* different allergens from where you were first tested, you may need to be retested.

Helpful hint 1: There is no particular benefit in automatically repeating skin or blood tests every year.

Helpful hint 2: Skin and blood tests do not indicate when you can stop allergy immunizing injections without worrying about a relapse.

Helpful hint 3: Three situations where it is useful to retest for allergy sensitivities are: if many years have passed, if you have moved to an area with significantly different allergens, or if your pattern of symptoms has changed.

Allergy Injections for Foods

Dr. Harold Nelson directed a study to immunize people who are allergic to peanuts. Most of the time you can avoid peanuts. But young children may be given a cookie or candy and even adults may eat at a restaurant where peanut is a contaminant of or is added to a particular food. Since peanut allergy can cause fatal reactions, doctors view peanut allergy more seriously than simple hayfever. Immunizing a person would give extra protection in case of an inadvertent ingestion.

Fatal peanut allergy is an extreme example of an allergic reaction. But people with less severe reactions often ask for immunizing injections to foods so they can eat whatever they want.

Dr. Nelson's study showed that most of the peanut injections were tolerated and that sensitivity to peanut was reduced. However, thirty-five percent of the injections resulted in a *generalized* reaction that had to be treated with emergency medicine. Furthermore, the doctors were so afraid of the terrible consequences of a fatal anaphylactic allergic reaction that they were afraid to feed these people peanuts to test whether the injections actually protected against fatal reactions. They were very aware that similar provocative tests performed in other research laboratories had resulted in several fatalities.

So, my word of advice is to forget about injections for food allergy. Just avoid the food. And for occasions when you inadvertently eat a food you are allergic to, carry and know how to use an emergency kit that your doctor can prescribe. The two common ones are Ana-Kit and Epi-pen.

Helpful hint 1: If you are allergic to a food, avoid the food.

Helpful hint 2: Don't participate in a study where doctors are trying to immunize you for food allergy. Let others be the guinea pigs.

Helpful hint 3: Carry and know how to use an emergency kit for sudden allergic reactions to foods.

14

Alternative Treatments, Multiple Chemical Sensitivity, Chronic Fatigue Syndrome, Fibromyalgia, Clinical Ecology

Traditional medicine is practiced by doctors who learn medicine at university medical schools in the United States and Canada. They examine diseases using objective measurements, controlled tests, laborious research, and what at times seems like unnecessary skepticism and doubt about a treatment until the treatment has been subjected to exhaustive "scientific analysis".

Alternative medicine is practiced by health care professionals who learn from a variety of sources including Eastern practitioners, Europeans, Shamans, Indians, and self-taught individuals. It includes a potpourri of disciplines such as acupuncture, herbalism, orthomolecular belief, Indian ayurveda, chiropractic, osteopathy, homeopathy, aromatherapy, massage, meditation, yoga, hypnotism, and Christian Science, to name a few of the more common practices.

It may surprise you to learn that traditional and alternative health care professionals share a trait. Although practitioners of a particular discipline may have trained in the same way, and even in the same school, each individual usually adopts his or her own style. Thus a particular chiropractor, homeopathist, and yoga master won't prescribe exactly the same treatment as another. Nor does each traditional doctor think exactly alike.

To make this even more complicated, some practitioners combine treatments. For example, treatment for high blood pressure may combine exercise, biofeedback, and a "traditional" antihypertensive drug. Treatment for being overweight may combine exercise, a low calorie diet, and a program of self-hypnosis. Treatment for chronic pain may combine acupuncture, an anti-inflammatory medication, and an antidepressant.

Thus medical care, whether traditional or alternative, is a pallette of options where *you and your doctor* must figure out what is best for *you*.

Like all diseases allergy has its share of "alternative" options. This chapter discusses most of them. Scientific studies show that alternative treatments, while they help certain *select* individuals are less reliable than traditional methods. However, traditional methods aren't perfect either, and one of the alternatives may work for you.

The sections of this chapter tell you what we know about acupuncture, homeopathy, yoga, hypnosis, chiropractic, herbalism, vitamin C, bee pollen, ion generators, Ma Huang, Chemical Sensitivity, Chronic Fatigue, Fibromyalgia, Clinical Ecology, and Monday Morning Sickness.

Acupuncture for Asthma

Needling the Ding Chuan point can relieve airway obstruction. In a study performed on Danish subjects a few lucky patients obtained about twenty percent improvement in air flow. Unfortunately the Danish study was the most successful of the controlled acupuncture studies. The uncontrolled studies cannot be considered because there is no way to compare results.

Helpful hint 1: Properly done acupuncture can provide about twenty percent relief in certain asthmatics.

Helpful hint 2: When acupuncture works, it needs to be repeated frequently because acupuncture is not a cure.

Helpful hint 3: Before you get your hopes up that you will respond to acupuncture, you need to know that traditional medicine achieves seventy-five to eighty percent improvement in symptoms. This would be a much better bet to help you.

Homeopathy for Allergy and Asthma

Homeopathy is based on the principle that you can counteract toxic substances in your body by ingesting those substances in dilute form. Actually, in classic homeopathy, you don't even ingest the substance. Instead you ingest a mirror of the substance.

To prepare classic homeopathic medicine, you dilute the substance such as a food or a pollen many, many times. Each time you dilute the substance, you tap the outside of the container to realign the molecules, a process called succussion. In the end you are said to have none of the molecules of food or pollen in the container. Instead you have water molecules that have taken on the shape of the food or pollen. These "mirrors" of molecules are what you swallow.

Some homeopathic doctors merely dilute the offending substances to very weak doses and don't try to achieve the "mirror" effect.

You may purchase homeopathic remedies in health food stores and specialty supermarkets.

A study from Scotland showed certain hayfever and asthma sufferers felt better after homeopathic treatment. However, when doctors measured the patients' nasal and lung function to determine *how much* the patients had improved, the doctors couldn't detect a measurable change.

Helpful hint 1: Certain people feel better when they use a homeopathic remedy even though objective tests don't detect a change in the underlying disease.

Yoga, Hypnosis, and The Power Of Suggestion for Allergy and Asthma

Yoga, hypnosis, and suggestion are forms of mental relaxation and physical control. Pranayama is a specific form of yoga for respiration.

In one asthma study a few subjects improved fifty percent. This was a temporary effect, but it obviosuly helped these people.

Helpful hint 1: Hypnosis, yoga, and other relaxation techniques have been shown to help select individuals.

Helpful hint 2: Relaxation techniques work best when combined with avoidance of allergens, using traditional medication for temporary relief, and, when indicated, taking allergy injections to build your immunity.

Osteopathy and Chiropractic

Osteopathy can run the gamut from a traditional medical doctor who graduates a school of osteopathy, takes a traditional residency, and practices traditional medicine to a doctor who is more like a chiropractor.

Chiropractic believes that the key to illness is in the alignment of the spine. While spinal alignment is important for musculo-skeletal problems, controlled studies haven't shown that liver disease, arthritis, asthma, hayfever, cancer, and so forth are due to spinal problems even though many chiropractors treat these conditions.

Nevertheless, there are people who feel better after chiropractic treatment. When it comes to allergy and asthma, the number who feel better are few and far between when you examine the results of treatment with a controlled study. If you merely ask allergic people how they feel after a form of treatment like chiropractic (and if you don't care what the objective data shows) you will find any kind of treatment may help a few select individuals because the pollen count, exposure to dust, and the ability to cope varies from day to day. If you catch a person on the right day, you will obtain a good report. This could coincide with a treatment and lead to the false conclusion that the treatment helped.

Helpful hint 1: Chiropractic has not been shown to be a reliable treatment for allergy and asthma even though once in awhile certain people feel better when they take chiropractic treatments.

Helpful hint 2: Even if chiropractic makes you feel better with a chronic disease such as allergy, you should see a doctor to find out if traditional treatment has something to offer too.

Herbalism

Herbalism is the science of finding, growing, and using herbs for the health and welfare of mankind. Verro Tyler, a professor at Purdue University and an expert on the subject of herbalism, divides herbalism into true and false herbalism.

True herbalism

According to Professor Tyler, true herbalism is the practice of testing herbs scientifically, reporting on the results honestly, producing herbs ethically, and using herbs wisely.

False Herbalism

False herbalism is practiced by people who preach the following philosophy.

•The pharmaceutical industry is a gang of companies who conspire to hide the true value of herbs from the general public.
•Herbs can do no harm to human beings.
•Whole herbs are more effective than the chemicals that are found in and can be isolated from herbs.
•Organically grown herbs are superior to synthetic drugs.
•Herbs have the power to cure people miraculously.

Dr. Tyler who is a stickler for the truth is familiar with the arguments of false herbalists. He points out that contrary to what false herbalists say the pharmaceutical industry invests a great deal of time and money to find herbs with medicinal value. Companies recognize that herbs can be valuable, and they send botanists to rain forests, jungles, and mountain tops throughout the world hoping that the botanists will find clues to new drugs that will cure diseases.

In fact, many of our most effective drugs have come from plants. For example, aspirin comes from the bark of the willow tree and digitalis comes from the foxglove plant.

To the charge that herbs can do no harm, Dr. Tyler explains that herbs *can* do harm. The herb comfrey contains allantoin. This promotes wound healing. However comfrey also contains carcinogenic alkaloids. In other words, like most drugs and chemicals there is a good and bad side to herbs.

To the assertion that organically grown herbs are best, Dr. Tyler explains that organically grown has come to mean that *no* chemical fertilizers or pesticides are used. However plants cannot grow without fertilizer and chemicals such as nitrogen, phosphorus and potassium. These must already *be in* or *brought to* the soil in which the plant is growing. Whether the farmer brings chemicals in a bag or takes advantage of the fertilizers that are already in the soil is moot. Either way, plants need "fertilizer" to grow.

Finally, Dr. Tyler explains that each anecdotal story about a person who was cured by herbs needs to be proven in a *controlled* study. Even if true, you need to ask how many people had to be treated with this method to find the one that could be cured.

Helpful hint 1: Proponents of true herbalism are on the right track because true herbalism can lead to helpful health care.

Helpful hint 2: Proponents of false herbalism create mistrust and suspicion. They prevent true herbalists from conducting the kind of rigorous scientific studies necessary to show that herbs can be useful.

How Vitamin C Was Thought To Help Allergies

You may have heard miraculous claims for vitamin C. Those who support its virtues say it can prevent colds, cancer, and allergies, to name a few of the benefits that have been reported.

In the case of allergy, vitamin C has been known to reduce the histamine level in the bloodstream. This may make vitamin C sound potentially helpful until I tell you that there isn't much histamine in your bloodstream. Most of your body's histamine is contained within Mast cells and Basophils which don't release their histamine into the blood stream unless they are forced to do so by IgE and allergen reacting together. Nevertheless, if histamine *was* in your bloodstream, vitamin C could reduce its level.

Dr. Harold Nelson was curious about the rumor that vitamin C could alleviate allergy. So he fed vitamin C to allergic volunteers and measured their symptoms. He also tested their skin sensitivity before and after they ingested vitamin C. Despite ingesting 2,000 milligrams of vitamin C a day, the skin tests and symptoms did not change.

As you read previously, *many* chemical mediators contribute to the allergic reaction. So even though vitamin C can lower the histamine level in the blood, this only reduces *one* of the multiple chemical mediators that cause allergic reactions.

Helpful hint 1: When you hear a scientist advocate that a complex disease like allergy can be treated by a single vitamin, you must make a superhuman effort not to be seduced by the simplicity of the proposal.

Helpful hint 2: Although vitamin C can lower the histamine level in your bloodstream, this doesn't have any effect on allergy symptoms or skin tests.

Helpful hint 3: Allergy sufferers have had a lot of disappointments over the years from eager salespeople who claim they have discovered a miraculous cure.

How Vitamin B1 Caused Allergy

Vitamins are supposed to make you healthy and strong. And they do. However, Dr. M. Fernandez, a doctor who practices in Spain, treated a woman who developed itching all over, swelling of the lips, and a drop in blood pressure when she took vitamin B1.

This woman was sorry she had ever heard of vitamin B1.

Helpful hint 1: In an earlier chapter you learned that a constituent of vitamin tablets can cause allergic reactions. Now you have learned that the vitamin itself can cause an allergic reaction.

Helpful hint 2: I hope you don't become paranoid and start thinking you aren't safe anywhere, but there is truth to the idea that life has dangers in unexpected places.

Helpful hint 3: Vitamin therapy for allergy may sound plausible, but in this case vitamins made a person worse.

Surprising Death From Bee Pollen

This is a scary story about an alternative method of treating allergy.

Certain people claim that ingesting bee pollen can cure allergy. Although there are no proven cases to confirm this, many people use bee pollen in the hope they'll get lucky.

My attitude used to be that it was anyone's constitutional right to take bee pollen if he wished. If he felt better, this was a good outcome since he wasn't harming himself, a kind of placebo effect, if you want to think of it that way.

Now, I've changed my mind. Two people had severe allergic reactions and died after using bee pollen. Bee pollen contains pollen from plants. If you ingest substances to which you are allergic, you can suffer a massive allergic reaction. What would you expect from purposely ingesting an uncontrolled, unmodified dose of the very substance that you are allergic to?

In this particular instance, two people were needlessly killed by bee pollen.

Helpful hint 1: If you are allergic to plant pollens, avoid bee pollen.

Helpful hint 2: There is no convincing research that shows ingesting bee pollen alleviates allergies.

Negative Ion Generators For Treating Asthma

If you purchase an ion generator, don't expect it to help your asthma. A lot of people have already made this costly mistake. Their ion generators sit idly in their closets. The idea that ion generators could help asthma came about when people noticed that their asthma was worse when there was the kind of atmospheric turbulence that creates ions in the air.

As a result of this theory an industry sprang up to manufacture ion generators that could counteract the effect of atmospherically-produced ions. Whether the theory was true or not, no one seemed to know or care. Dr. Harold Nelson, who doesn't like unsubstantiated theories, decided he had better study ion generators before the matter got out of hand.

Without disclosing what he was doing, Dr. Nelson exposed asthmatic volunteers to negative and positive ions. The ions didn't affect his volunteers one way or the other. They weren't worse, and they weren't better.

Helpful hint 1: Asthma symptoms can flare when the weather changes. But the increased symptoms patients experience are not due to ions in the air. There is another reason which doctors must still figure out.

Helpful hint 2: Ion generators won't make your asthma better or worse.

Helpful hint 3: Whenever there's a theory in medicine, someone, somewhere, will invent a machine to exploit the theory whether or not the theory has a basis in fact.

Ma Huang, Unsafe at Any Speed

The United States Food and Drug Administration has always had a program to monitor the side effects of prescription drugs. Over the past few years, though, the FDA added another program called MEDWATCH. This monitors the side effects *non-prescription* medications and led to the discovery that Chinese Ephedra (Ephedrica sinica), which is the active ingredient in the herb Ma Huang, caused several deaths.

Ma Huang is a traditional herb that is found in teas and homeopathic remedies that are sold to treat allergy, aid in weight loss, and provide increased energy. Death was, of course, the most serious side effect. Other side effects of Chinese ephedra were nervousness, tremor, headaches, chest pain, heart attack, psychosis, and seizures.

Helpful hint 1: Over-the-counter herbs, teas, and homeopathic remedies can cause serious side effects. They need to be used with caution.

Helpful hint 2: In one sense, over-the-counter preparations are probably more dangerous than prescription medicines. Because they are sold over-the-counter, we often assume they are perfectly safe even though we may have doubts about whether they will do any good. With the attitude that 'I have nothing to lose', you might be tempted to try some of these preparations. This was a fatal mistake for several people. The reason I say that prescription medicines may be safer is that we know they are powerful, treat them with respect, and only take them when necessary.

Condurango Bark And Latex Allergy

Dr. Bernhard Przybilla from Germany reported that condurango bark, which is a remedy for stomachaches and an ingredient in certain bitter drinks, can cause asthma, hives, and swelling of the body. He treated a nurse who was allergic to latex and reacted after drinking a tea with condurango bark extract in it.

The poor nurse who already had enough problems dealing with latex allergy at work, now has to be careful about what he (Yes, this was a male nurse.) can eat.

Helpful hint 1: Cross reactions between seemingly unrelated substances make allergy dangerous and scary. Cross reaction is the technical term that indicates that two substances that *appear* unrelated contain an identical molecular substance that can cause an allergic reaction.

The Latest Word About Multiple Chemical Sensitivity, Chronic Fatigue, and Fibromyalgia

Over the past few years, the disease chronic fatigue syndrome has hit the headlines of nearly every newspaper, magazine, and radio-doc show in America. The usual symptoms are fatigue, sleep disturbances, memory loss, depression, difficulty thinking, headache, and sore throat.

If you think about it a moment, these symptoms are common and affect all of us at one time or another. So the question is when do you diagnose chronic fatigue and when do you blame the flu, an infection, depression, family quarrels, a bad night's sleep, or a bad day at the office?

The usual clue was when the symptoms persisted for weeks and months and when your doctors couldn't find a more serious condition like hormone imbalance, cancer, or heart disease.

To the rescue came the National Institutes of Health which spent a lot of money to study chronic fatigue. The doctors came up with a list of eleven symptoms and three physical changes that other doctors could use to diagnose these baffling illnesses. However, when the list was put to the test, doctors discovered that many chronic fatigue, multiple chemical sensitivity, and fibromyalgia patients didn't have *consistent* physical changes. So the National Institutes of Health doctors removed physical changes from the list. They then had to eliminate positive laboratory tests because the patients didn't have *consistent* positive tests, either.

By the time the National Institutes' doctors finished fine-tuning their advice, they had to conclude that doctors in private practice had to rely on their patients' histories to make the diagnosis. So, if a patient reported he had chronic fatigue symptoms (or multiple chemical sensitivity or fibromyalgia) they had the disease.

Having a patient diagnose his own illness based on how he feels is a new and unique way to diagnose medical illness! Usually diagnosis is the doctor's job after listening to the history, finding objective changes on physical examination, and obtaining laboratory tests that confirm the diagnosis.

To make matters more confusing, the symptoms of chronic fatigue are similar to the symptoms found in multiple chemical sensitivity, fibromyalgia, reactions to silicone breast implants, environmental illness, the Twentieth Century Syndrome, and Candida Syndrome. These conditions don't have characteristic physical changes or particular and consistent abnormal laboratory tests, either.

Dr. Dedra Buchwald from Harborview Medical Center and Dr. Deborah Garrity of Washington University School of Medicine became interested in these conditions since certain experts felt allergy and an altered immune system caused them.

To begin, the doctors selected thirty patients with known chronic fatigue, multiple chemical sensitivity, and fibromyalgia. Since there were thirty with each diagnosis (ninety people in all), they thought they would be able to figure out which symptoms characterized which illness.

After reviewing the histories, physical examinations, and laboratory tests of each person, the doctors found all ninety had fatigue, fever, sore throats, headaches, swollen or tender lymph nodes, joint pains, muscle aches, muscle weakness, sleep disturbances, hoarseness, burning in the nose and mouth, itching or irritated skin, memory loss, forgetfulness, confusion, clouded thoughts, irritability, and feeling depressed. Studies of the blood and urine were normal. Special tests for hormones, viruses, including Epstein-Barr virus (EBV), and X-rays were similar, too.

The doctors were puzzled. There was no way to determine which patient had which disease. They couldn't explain how these patients had been divided into three groups in the first place. And like other researchers before them, they weren't able to determine the underlying cause, except to say that allergy might have been a *contributing* factor in a few cases.

Doctors Buchwald and Garrity were also interested in what type of health care professional got the best treatment results. After all, patients aren't fussy about what name we doctors call an illness as long as they get better. Unfortunately very few patients felt better and none had been cured even though they had consulted a wide variety of specialists including environmental physicians, clinical ecologists, allergists, medical doctors, chiropractors, naturopaths, homeopaths, psychiatrists, psychologists, acupuncturists, and massage therapists. Thus, Drs. Garrity and Buchwald concluded that doctors, whether they practice traditional, alternative, or anything in-between, can't distinguish between these conditions nor can they treat them successfully. This reflects our ignorance of what causes these illnesses.

So if you have the above symptoms or have been diagnosed with one of these conditions, modern medicine doesn't know what they are, what causes them, what cures them, or even how to distinguish one from the other. The best approach is to seek relief from the symptoms as best you can.

Helpful hint 1: Facing the fact that modern science can't cure all diseases is discouraging. But it is best to face the facts than have false, unrealistic hopes.

Helpful hint 2: If you suffer from the debilitating symptoms described above, your diagnosis will likely depend on what type of health care professional you consult. Clinical ecologists tend to diagnose yeast syndrome or multiple chemical sensitivity, allergists tend to diagnose allergy, internists tend to diagnose fibromyalgia, family doctors may diagnose Lyme disease, and so forth. Nevertheless the illnesses seem identical based on history, absence of physical changes, and lack of characteristic laboratory tests.

Helpful hint 3: If you have been diagnosed with any of these conditions, fight like hell to get your doctor to change the diagnosis. Ask them to run whatever tests they can think of. Even consider consulting a therapist about possible mild depression. Since there are no physical changes or abnormal laboratory tests and therefore no treatment for these conditions, you are better off doing whatever you can to look for an illness we do know how to treat than going along with a diagnosis of chronic fatigue which no one knows anything about.

Helpful hint 4: The best approach to these baffling conditions is to undertake a systematic trial of various treatments, follow a healthy diet, and force yourself to exercise regularly. I wish I could be more helpful and hopeful.

Total Environmental Allergy And Clinical Ecology

Physicians who practice Clinical Ecology or Environmental Medicine have identified a group of symptoms they call Total Environmental Allergy or Twentieth Century Syndrome. The people who suffer from this disease are said to be allergic to the chemicals we are all exposed to at work and home.

Dr. Abba Terr who is at Stanford University Medical School investigated fifty cases where people had been told they had Total Environmental Allergy. He found nineteen of them had no disease or just a common condition such as asthma, hepatitis, conjunctivitis, or hyperventilation.

The remaining thirty-one patients had numerous complaints, but their physical examination, blood, urine, and x-ray tests were normal. There was no defect or even a minor deficiency in their immune system. These were cases where the only evidence of an illness was in the history.

Despite the absence of abnormalities, all fifty patients were following a treatment their ecologist had prescribed. They were avoiding plastic and synthetic materials at home and work, had moved to the country, were observing restrictive diets, and in some cases were taking allergy injections. Unbelievably, eight of the fifty patients who were following their ecologist's instructions had *no* symptoms before they even began following their ecologist's instructions. So of course they had no symptoms afterwards.

In the final analysis, Dr. Terr found that eight patients had no symptoms to begin with. The remaining forty-two who did have symptoms were no better after treatment. Thus, except for the eight who weren't complaining anyway, the rest had not improved.

Helpful hint 1: Total Environmental Allergy was a new idea. New ideas shouldn't be discouraged. Otherwise doctors would never learn anything. However, a new idea shouldn't be believed until it has been scrutinized carefully using controlled studies and *only* after the theory has been shown to be correct. In this case the theory has been shown to be incorrect except in a few rare instances.

Helpful hint 2: Some patients may benefit from avoidance of synthetic and plastic materials. This makes great headlines and is fun to read about in newspapers and magazines, but the problem is greatly exaggerated.

Helpful hint 3: One way to have good treatment results is to begin with people who are asymptomatic, give them a treatment, and measure their response. This type of patient is an ideal candidate for uncontrolled research. He will always report good results.

Monday Morning Sickness and Workplace Allergy

You may have heard of the condition Monday-Morning Blues which begins upon going to work after a relaxing weekend. Now, allergists have discovered Monday-Morning Flu's.

A group of doctors were confronted with patients who developed flu-like symptoms every Monday morning. At first they thought this must be an allergic reaction caused by something in the workplace. They looked high and low but found nothing. Then they realized they should think of other possibilities besides allergy.

Upon investigating the air-conditioning system at their patients' workplaces, the doctors found bacteria had grown in the ventilation ducts over the weekend and had produced toxic byproducts which entered the air when the system was turned on Monday morning. Decontaminating the vents stopped the symptoms.

Helpful hint 1: Although symptoms which occur at the same time and place usually indicate allergy, there are exceptions to this rule.

Helpful hint 2: Cases of chemical sensitivity or chemical allergy sometimes have a logical and mundane explanation.

15

Insect-Sting Allergy

Bee stings can cause death in highly allergic individuals. This makes stinging-insect allergy a major concern to allergists. We spend a lot of time diagnosing and treating patients to prevent needless fatalaties.

When bees sting, they inject about ten different chemicals. Some of the chemicals are toxic and cause pain, redness, swelling, and itching *at the site* of the sting. If the stinger is dirty, an infection can develop *at the site* of the sting. These are *local* reactions. They may even persist for several days. But no matter how large, swollen, or uncomfortable you are, a reaction that is limited to the site of the sting is a *local* reaction.

On the other hand, if you develop symptoms *far away* from the sting, you are having a *systemic* (or anaphylactic) reaction. These are the dangerous ones. You can break out in hives and have an attack of asthma. In extreme cases you can have fatal shock.

Those who are truly allergic should undertake a series of immunizing injections to protect against fatal bee sting allergy.

The first study explains how to determine how long you need to take immunizing injections to obtain permanent protection against stinging insects. The second study unmasks myths about killer bees which are terrorizing certain parts of the United States, and the third study tells you how fast you must remove a honeybee's stinger.

Bee Sting Injections Need Not Last Forever

In 1979 there was a mini-revolution in treating bee sting allergy. For many years Dr. Mary Loveless had pleaded with allergists to inject bee venom instead of whole-body extract when treating bee sting allergy. Most of the medical community ignored her because whole-body extract had the advantage of being easier to make, less expensive to give, and seemed to be as effective as venom.

After spending hundreds of hours reviewing the old studies and after several years of performing new studies, doctors at Johns Hopkins Hospital discovered that Dr. Loveless had been right. Venom was superior. Therefore, despite venom's higher cost, allergists started using venom.

Treatments begin with approximately twenty injections to build the immunity to a protective level. This is generally followed by monthly injections to maintain the immunity. At first no one knew how long the immunity would last. So the injections were recommended indefinitely.

Then Drs. Robert Reisman and Martin Valentine discovered that you do not have to continue bee venom shots forever. Most children can stop after three years. Adults usually need about five years. Don't stop injections on your own, though. Consult your allergist who will help you figure out when it is appropriate for you to stop immunizing bee-sting injections.

Remember, too, that people who experience *local* reactions don't need treatment at all. The definition of bee-sting allergy is a *systemic* reaction. In other words, you react someplace other than where you were stung. When you swell up horribly or have a lot of pain at the site of the sting, this is not allergy in the medical sense. To be allergic, you must break out in hives, have asthma, have trouble swallowing, or collapse. Local itching, swelling, and pain don't count.

After taking your medical history, if your allergist is still not sure whether you are allergic, he can figure it out by doing skin tests for bee venom.

Helpful hint 1: You have the best chance for achieving a permanent cure for bee-sting allergy if you start injection treatment when you are young.

Helpful hint 2: Each case of bee-sting treatment must be evaluated *individually* before deciding when to stop a series of immunizing injections.

Helpful hint 3: Bee-sting allergy refers to *generalized* or *systemic* reactions, not to local, toxic, or bacterial reactions which occur at the site of the sting.

Killer Bee Threat Is Overdramatized

Newspaper editors love a good scary story. The fact that killer bees have invaded the United States is made for their headlines.

Killer bees are bees that originally came from outside the United States. They are bigger and more aggressive than domestic bees. When angry, they sting in swarms instead of one at a time.

But do they kill? And do they cause allergic reactions? This isn't a science fiction story where a single-genetically altered bee goes on a rampage and terrorizes the population. Doctors estimate it would take nearly 1,000 simultaneous stings to kill a human. This number of stings at one time is extremely unlikely.

What makes killer bees terrifying is they fly in groups, get angry easily, and sting in swarms. When it comes to possible allergy to killer bees, they are actually *less* dangerous than domestic bees. Dr. J. E. Lowry measured killer-bee venom sacs and found that they contain less venom than domestic bees. Since allergic reactions depend, to some extent, on the amount of allergen entering your body, it would be *less* likely for a *single* killer bee to cause a fatal reaction than a *single* domestic bee.

Helpful hint 1: In allergy, the larger the dose of allergens you receive, the worse your reaction. Since killer bees have less venom than domestic bees, you have less chance of a severe *allergic* reaction from killer bees than from domestic bees.

Helpful hint 2: Stay away from killer bees. They are mean and ornery.

Remove the Stinger Fast

Dr. Michael Schumacher timed how fast a honeybee's venom sac empties. This may sound like frivolous research, but it has important implications.

When a bee stings, the stinger and venom sac are torn from the bee's body. Over the next few seconds the sac pumps itself dry. So the sooner you remove the stinger, the less venom you get.

Unfortunately Dr. Schumacher's study showed that it only takes about five seconds for the sac to empty. So you've got to be lightning fast to get the stinger out.

Helpful hint 1: Don't waste time yelling and cursing when a honeybee stings you. Take the stinger out immediately. Then you can yell and curse.

Helpful hint 2: Sometimes allergists tell their patients to do things that are next to impossible like be cool and calm when a honeybee stings you so you can pull the honeybee stinger out in less than five seconds.

16

Penicillin and Drug Allergy

Drug reactions are increasingly common in modern medicine. Statistics show nearly ten percent of hospitalized patients experience a reaction to one of the drugs they are given. Outside the hospital the figures are just as bad. They are worse if you include over-the-counter drugs.

Pick a medication. Any medication you can think of. Sad to say, there are none that can be guaranteed one-hundred percent safe from side effects.

In this chapter, you will learn about allergic-type reactions. You may want to re-read the section on *adverse* drug reactions because allergic reactions are only one kind of reaction you can have from a drug. The others are intolerance, metabolic, idiosyncratic, overdose, and pharmacologic.

Possibly the most commonly diagnosed allergic reaction is the reaction to the antibiotic penicillin. Since penicillin is such an important antibiotic, doctors have devoted a great deal of time to studying what causes penicillin reactions and how to avoid them. This has provided us with our basic understanding of all drug reactions. What you will read about penicillin applies to every kind of drug allergy.

You will read three studies about penicillin. The first describes how doctors can prescribe penicillin to a penicillin-allergic patient without fear of an allergic reaction. The second describes a test to detect penicillin allergy. The third study explains why massive screening of the general population for penicillin allergy would not be useful.

Penicillin Allergy No Longer A Widespread Problem

If you have been *told* you are allergic to penicillin, there are six ways for you to take penicillin anyway without fear of an allergic reaction.

1. Dr. Dorothy Sogn reported that most people who have been told they are allergic to penicillin are not *really* allergic to it. She took histories, did examinations, and tested patients who claimed they were sensitive. She discovered that seventy-five percent had been misdiagnosed. Thus, most people who think they are allergic to penicillin are not truly allergic and have no reason to fear penicillin.

2. The second way to take penicillin is a simple bit of wisdom. Use *another* antibiotic. There are many antibiotics which kill bacteria effectively. You aren't wedded to penicillin. Of course, a corollary of this rule is: Don't use *any* antibiotic unless you *truly* need it. The more often you use an antibiotic the greater the chance you may wind up becoming allergic to it.

3. If you absolutely need penicillin, but are allergic to it, your doctor can treat you beforehand with anti-allergy

medicines. This can prevent a reaction or at least reduce its intensity.

4. If you have a particular infection where nothing but penicillin will work, such as in certain infections of the heart or bones, you can take penicillin intravenously in gradually increasing doses until you reach the amount that kills the bacteria (the therapeutic level). This *desensitizes* you so you don't react. This needs to be done by a trained physician in a hospital where you can be observed and monitored continuously.

5. Dr. M.J. Torres from Spain found that certain patients react to penicillin-like drugs when the drugs are given orally but not when given intravenously. This shows that in some individuals the *route* the drug is given makes a difference between having and not having an allergic reaction.

6. Finally, Dr. Barbara Stark figured out a dosing schedule to desensitize patients orally instead of intravenously. As with intravenous desensitization, you need to be strictly monitored during the process. Don't try this on your own.

Helpful hint 1: The majority of people who think they are allergic to penicillin are not allergic to penicillin.

Helpful hint 2: If you are truly allergic to penicillin, you can usually take the drug after a simple desensitization procedure.

Helpful hint 3: Do not take antibiotics (or any other drug) unnecessarily.

Helpful hint 4: If you are desensitized to penicillin, this is not a lifetime cure. Desensitization must be repeated every time you need to use penicillin.

Tests for Penicillin Allergy

Dr. Louis Mendelson from Connecticut solved a knotty problem in penicillin allergy. When allergists test for penicillin allergy, they must use two different chemicals. One of them, called Minor Determinant Mixture, is unstable.

Strictly speaking, Minor Determinant Mixture is supposed to be made fresh according to a particular process. However some doctors make a low-priced copy by placing penicillin in an alkaline solution at room temperature. Although penicillin breaks down under these conditions, the products aren't exactly identical to Minor Determinant Mixture. When used for testing, this material is about sixty-five percent accurate. The scientifically-made mixture is ninety-five percent accurate.

Dr. Mendelson and his co-workers developed a freeze-dried Minor Determinant Mixture. Freeze-drying protects the potency and allows the scientifically-made material to be shipped anywhere. A doctor who used this freeze-dried Minor Determinant Mixture would be able to tell you your *exact* chance of having penicillin allergy.

Helpful hint 1: If you have been tested for penicillin allergy, ask if both Major and Minor Determinant Mixtures were used.

Helpful hint 2: If Minor Determinant Mixture was used, ask whether your doctors made it themselves. If the mixture was made by your doctors, the results are only sixty-five percent accurate.

Helpful hint 3: A drug company is trying to manufacture freeze-dried Minor Determinant Mixture so it will be available to all doctors throughout the United States.

Testing For Penicillin Allergy Has Limited Value

The availability of chemicals that test for penicillin allergy makes testing all of us sound like a good idea. We would know our level of sensitivity, and those of us who aren't allergic wouldn't have to worry. Those who are allergic could take precautions. However, Dr. Timothy Sullivan showed that *routine* population-wide testing would probably be a waste of time.

While it's true that Major and Minor Determinant Mixtures show allergy with high degree of accuracy, the tests don't tell the future. The more penicillin you use, the greater the chance you can become allergic. You would have to be re-tested each time you wanted to use penicillin to make sure you had not converted between the time you were previously tested and the present time.

Helpful hint 1: Testing for penicillin allergy is accurate when the correct test materials are used.

Helpful hint 2: Testing for penicillin allergy determines a person's state of sensitivity *at the moment in time the test is performed.* The tests are not crystal balls and do not predict or guarantee that you won't become allergic in the future.

Helpful hint 3: Despite what I just said, when Minor Determinant Mixture becomes available there will be extensive testing for penicillin allergy. People who test negative will believe in their non-allergic status and not realize that, over time, they might become allergic. This false assumption may make them complacent about taking penicillin when, in fact, each of us must be careful no matter what drug we take and no matter how many times in the past we have used that drug without difficulty.

Helpful hint 4: Allergy tests only disclose the *current* degree of sensitivity. They do not predict the future.

Helpful hint 5 Sometimes our wishful thinking overwhelms our common sense.

17

Allergy and Pregnancy

Pregnancy is a time when a woman's body undergoes major changes. It should come as no surprise, then, that allergies may change, too. Allergy can begin, stay the same, become worse, or even improve. There is no test to predict which way allergy will go in a particular case. The first study discusses this issue.

The next two studies explain that allergy injections do not harm the fetus. They may even immunize the unborn child.

Asthma Symptoms During Pregnancy

Allergists and obstetricians know that pregnancy can aggravate nasal allergies and asthma. This does not happen to all women or even to most women, but it is not *uncommon* either.

Dr. Michael Schatz surveyed over 300 allergic women and found that the outlook is not as bad as many people had imagined. Most women who suffer from allergy have the same level of symptoms during pregnancy as before they became pregnant. Of the remainder, a few get better, and a few get worse. Of those who become worse, seventy-five percent revert to their original level after they deliver. Only twenty-five percent remain worse.

Thus, when pregnancy triggers asthma or when pre-existing asthma becomes worse, this is usually only a *temporary* situation.

> **Helpful hint 1**: There is no need to panic if your asthma becomes worse when you are pregnant. There is a good chance your symptoms will subside after you deliver.

> **Helpful hint 2**: Asthma sometimes improves during pregnancy. Unfortunately, this is often only temporary.

Allergy Injections Don't Make The Fetus Allergic

Women who take allergy immunizing injections during pregnancy do not put their infants at risk for developing allergies, do not cause various diseases, do not raise the risk of congenital abnormalities, and do not cause difficult labor and delivery. If you think about it, this is what you would expect from an injection that does not contain drugs or foreign chemicals but is made from extracts of grasses, trees, weeds, pets, and dust which are substances that enter the body anyway.

On the other hand doctors are born worriers. Certain ones who worried more than most thought it would be a good idea to look at what happens to the fetus when the mother gets injections. To conduct a foolproof experiment, the doctors had to find women who were getting injections for something other than grasses, weeds, trees, and dust because they didn't want a skeptic arguing that a background pollen count or dust exposure corrupted the experiment and invalidated the findings.

Dr. David Graft and his colleagues found their candidate-subjects among a group of pregnant women who were receiving injections of honeybee venom. No one could say that extraneous honey bee venom contaminated or skewed the results because except for the injections, the women were not being stung by honeybees. The mothers had been found sensitive to honeybees and were receiving immunizing injections, which are described in a previous chapter under insect-sting allergy.

After the mothers delivered their babies, the doctors tested the infants and found that the infants were perfectly normal. They had suffered no ill effects and hadn't been sensitized to bee venom.

Previous studies had shown that allergy injections are safe for the mother. Dr. Graft's study showed that injections are safe for the fetus, too.

Helpful hint 1: Since allergy injections contain only natural substances (i.e. no drugs or medications) one would not think allergy injections would be harmful to the fetus or detrimental to pregnancy. Scientific studies confirm this.

Helpful hint 2: Sometimes doctors have to be very clever to set up the conditions for an experiment so that skeptics like me will be satisfied that the results are meaningful.

Fetus Protected Against Allergy When Mother Gets Shots

In another study, the previously mentioned Dr. Michael Schatz was one of a group of San Diego Kaiser Hospital doctors who studied newborns whose mothers had received allergy injections during pregnancy. He and his co-workers discovered that the mothers had transferred some of their immunity to the fetus. Although doctors already knew injections weren't harmful, this was the first report that showed injections could be helpful.

Before taking this study as gospel truth, you should wait for confirming evidence from other investigators. Nevertheless this is encouraging news.

Helpful hint 1: A mother's immunizing injections seem to bolster the immunity of the fetus.

18

Hives, Angioedema, and Eczema

Dermatologists are trained to diagnose and treat skin conditions. However, there are two skin conditions that allergists are trained to treat and one where they can assist the dermatologist.

The skin conditions allergists are specifically trained to treat are hives and angioedema. Hives are superficial swellings of the skin, like giant mosquito bites. Angioedema is swelling underneath the skin that looks like someone hit you but without the black and blue mark. The condition allergists *assist* with is eczema. This is peeling, scaling, itching, and redness that in *some* cases is due to allergy.

The following studies explain more about these bothersome, frustrating, nerve-wracking, and often itchy diseases.

Definition of Chronic Hives

Dr. Alan Kaplan has studied hives for most of his medical career. So he is considered a world-class authority, a kind of guru of hives. Previously, hives were defined as chronic when they persisted more than six weeks. Acute meant they lasted less than six weeks even though six weeks is a long time when you can't sleep at night due to itching and are scratching your skin raw during the day.

Now, Dr. Kaplan has determined that the six-week definition is misleading. Since proper treatment depends so much on correct diagnosis, allergists must change their thinking.

According to Dr. Kaplan, acute hives should refer to hives which last one or two hours, go away, and then come back in a different location on your body. Thus, it is *not how many weeks* you have hives that matters. It is how long each hive persists at its location on your body. So even if you have suffered with hives for months, your hives are *acute* if they move around a lot from place to place on your body. This is an important distinction for diagnostic and therapeutic purposes.

When hives remain in the *same* location for hours at a time, this is chronic hives, even if you have only been symptomatic for a few weeks.

This may seem like semantics to you, but the reason hives behave differently is due to the underlying cause. And knowing the underlying cause leads to more appropriate and effective treatment.

Helpful hint 1: Sometimes just changing the definition of an illness can help doctors better understand a disease process. And better understanding leads to more effective treatment.

Trigger Of Chronic Hives

Chronic hives and itching are extremely annoying. Many times the culprit cannot be found. So when scientists discover something new to look for, it is of great interest.

Dr. Anthony Kulczycki at Washington University Medical School reported several cases of hives and itching which he traced to the artificial sweetener aspartame (Nutrasweet). This type of reaction is very uncommon. But if you have hives or itching, consider stopping aspartame on a trial basis.

Drs. Frank Martell and Edward Buckley from North Carolina discovered patients may get hives and angioedema from aspirin, sulfite, or tartrazine dye. Dr. Ann Wanner found a patient whose angioedema stopped as soon as his doctors removed a kidney stone.

I could go on and on about rare cases where doctors eventually found the cause of chronic hives and angioedema-type swelling. Unfortunately, the majority of the time no matter how many tests are done and no matter how many cases I could report to you, the cause cannot be determined. This doesn't mean you and your doctors should stop looking. But at a certain point you need to say "No more tests" and concentrate on learning the *safest* way to treat the symptoms.

Helpful hint 1: Certain chemicals which are innocuous to the majority of the population can cause allergic reactions in select individuals.

Helpful hint 2: Although aspartame may provoke an allergic reaction in select individuals, there is no need to ban this substance. The majority of the population tolerates it with no ill effect. Using the same logic, there is no need to ban peanut butter even though a few unfortunate, highly peanut-sensitive individuals would die if they ate peanut butter.

Helpful hint 3: I am sorry to tell you this, but most cases of chronic hives and angioedema (i.e. swelling) cannot be solved.

Hives And Swelling During Exercise

Have you ever exercised and broken out in hives or gotten itchy? I know this sounds strange, but it happens to some people. These kinds of reactions have occurred for years, but soon after Dr. Albert Sheffer wrote about them in a medical journal, there was a rash (excuse the expression) of such cases.

Exercise reactions are a fascinating problem, especially when you consider how important we think exercise is in keeping us healthy. People with this exercise-induced allergy get hives, itching, asthma, and even collapse when their bodies become warm during vigorous athletics. What is truly unbelievable is that some of these patients only experience these reactions if they eat a specific food (it's a different food for different people) *before* they exercise. Even more strange is that some only suffer if they eat that particular food *after* they exercise. Would you believe that celery, which seems innocuous to me, was the offending food in several cases?

Treatments are available, but just the idea of such an illness is remarkable.

Helpful hint 1: If you experience unusual symptoms during or shortly after exercise, see your family doctor or better yet, consult an allergist.

Pizza, Pizza, Pizza

Dr. Lyndon Mansfield, who practices allergy in Arizona, reported on a child who had severe respiratory distress, wheezing, hives all over his body, and throat swelling after eating pepperoni pizza. The case is interesting because the child had previously eaten pepperoni pizza with no ill-effect. However, on one particular day the child ate pizza and immediately went outside to play in the park.

Dr. Mansfield and his associates showed that the combination of sodium nitrite in the pepperoni and the exposure to sunlight caused a photo-allergic reaction which resulted in an asthma attack. Until this episode the child had only experienced a few small hives on exposure to sunlight and hadn't had asthma from eating pizza.

Helpful hint 1: Don't eat pizza in the park.

Eczema And Dust Mites

Eczema is an annoying condition where the skin is red, itchy, dry, cracked, and generally all-around uncomfortable. Some people have this from birth. In some it begins later in life. In some it subsides as the person ages. In some it persists.

Often there is nothing that cures eczema. Massive doses of cortisone-steroids will alleviate the problem, but then there are those darn cortisone side effects. Usually patients need to learn good skin care from a dermatologist and follow the routine faithfully, especially when they are getting better. The tendency to slack off when the skin improves is a *big* mistake.

Allergists can sometimes help eczema. In certain people, foods or airborne allergens, such as pollen or dust mites, cause itching which causes scratching which causes infections, all of which makes the eczema ten times worse than it has to be.

If you have chronic eczema, consulting an allergist to find out if foods or airborne allergens are contributing to your eczema can pay off handsomely.

Helpful hint 1: If you suffer from eczema, you have nothing to lose and a lot to gain by consulting an allergist.

Helpful hint 2: When your eczema is under control, that is the time to be most diligent with your skin care.

19

New Diseases

Considering the fact that medical science is unlocking the secrets of DNA, creating wonderful new drugs, applying genetic engineering to conquer a myriad of diseases, inventing high-tech instruments, and on the trail of advances about which we can only speculate, it is surprising that doctors still discover something mundane like a new disease. So when I hear of a new disease, I wonder if it is really new or were we doctors too focused on advanced research to notice our patients had symptoms that fit a pattern and should have been recognized earlier if we had been paying attention?

I don't know the answer to this philosophical question. But I do know that we allergists are making every effort to pay attention to what you tell us, and we have "new" diseases to report. The following studies discuss several of them. If one of them sounds familiar to you, consult your doctor.

You will read how latex, men, exercise, various occupations (yes, it's finally been proven that you can be allergic to work!), the act of eating, eye drops, copy paper, x-ray contrast material, a particular kind of skin infection, and teflon can cause allergy.

Latex Allergy

It used to be that surgeons and surgical nurses were the only ones who wore latex gloves for protection. Now, the world has gone topsy-turvy and everyone is wearing them due to the human immune-deficiency virus (HIV). Laboratory workers, nurses, dentists, hygienists, and even custodians wear gloves to protect *them* from you and *you* from them. Dr. John Yunginger from Minnesotta reported that over six billion pairs of gloves are used in the United States each year!

In addition to latex gloves, there are many medical products and even everyday products like balloons and condoms that are made from latex.

This widespread use of latex has led to seven to ten percent of hospital workers becoming allergic to latex.

There are three types of reaction. Your skin can become red, dry, itchy and cracked. This is called contact dermatitis-type eczema. You can develop hives. This is called contact urticaria. Or you may develop asthma and shock. This is called anaphylaxis.

Once doctors realized what was happening, they noticed latex reactions explained a lot of problems that had been a mystery. Dr. Dennis Ownby of the Henry Ford Hospital reported that patients who were thought to react to barium used in x-ray studies actually reacted to the latex tubes used to inject the barium into the bowel. Dr. Francoise Porri found that a percentage of anesthetic reactions were really due to latex tubes used to administer the anesthetics. Even infant pacifiers can cause latex reactions.

At one time it was thought that talcum powder or corn starch which is used in latex gloves to make them easier to put on were responsible for these allergic reactions. Dr. Alexander Fisher, who is considered the dean of skin allergies, was skeptical and after a few experiments found that two chemicals in latex rubber (mercaptobenzothiazole and tetramethylthiuram) absorbed to corn starch and made it seem like the corn starch and talcum powder were the offending agents.

Dr. Fisher's work is interesting academically. But the lesson is the same either way: If your skin breaks out when you wear latex gloves, avoid latex. Dr. S. Tario showed even this may not be safe. Since latex absorbs to corn starch, everyone you work with may have to use non-latex gloves, too. Otherwise there is a chance that the corn starch that gets in the air from your co-workers' gloves will affect *you*.

Helpful hint 1: Latex allergy is a growing problem. And it will probably get worse.

Helpful hint 2: To avoid latex, you may have to enlist the cooperation of coworkers.

Testing For Latex Allergy Stretches The Truth

Dr. Lawrence Du Buske and a group of nine other doctors from around the world tested two hundred patients who said they were latex-sensitive. Doctor David Levy in France tested another group of patients consisting of sixty-five nurses who said they were latex-sensitive. Between the two studies, the doctors used three different blood tests, four different types of latex, and a popular latex skin test. The results were amazing. Combining all patients, the doctors found that the tests confirmed latex sensitivity in only about five percent of the subjects.

The doctors concluded that either most patients imagine they are sensitive or latex tests aren't adequate to the task. To find out which answer was true, the doctors asked many of the patients to wear the gloves they claimed were causing their symptoms. In this type of *direct-contact* test, *everyone* who had claimed they were sensitive developed a reaction.

Healthful hint 1: We have a lot to learn about how to test people for latex allergy. In the meantime, if you itch, wheeze, swell up, break out in hives, or have trouble breathing when you are exposed to latex, stay away from latex.

Healthful hint 2: Be careful if someone wants to *skin*-test you for latex. The skin tests aren't accurate, and besides that you may suffer an acute attack of asthma and need to be treated which is what happened to several patients in the above studies.

Healthful hint 3: Be skeptical if someone wants to test you for latex allergy using a *blood*-test. The results will likely be wrong, and this will lead you to a false conclusion.

Healthful hint 4: A good history is often more valuable than a high-tech test.

If You Are Allergic to Latex, Don't Eat Bananas

Dr. G. Safadi found that bananas contain a similar allergen to latex when he came upon a patient who developed asthma after eating bananas. As you know by now since you are almost finished with this book and about to become a full-fledged, card-carrying amateur allergist, this is called cross-reactivity.

Other doctors have shown that chestnuts, avocados, and ficus trees cross react with latex, too. Other foods that cross react with latex are papaya, avocado, kiwi, chestnut, wheat germ, and condurango bark which is found in certain herbal teas and bitter drinks.

Ragweed can also cross-react with latex.

Healthful hint 1: Latex allergy is a pervasive condition that can affect you in many ways.

Wife Allergic To Her Husband

Saying you are allergic to your wife or husband is a tired, old joke. However, allergists take everything seriously. Lo and behold, Dr. David Bernstein found several women who were truly allergic to their husbands.

In each case, the women broke out in hives, itched all over, and even had shortness of breath and wheezing minutes after having intercourse. Upon investigation, Dr. Bernstein found that the women had become allergic to their husband's sperm. After the diagnosis was confirmed by testing, Dr. Bernstein made a special serum, immunized the women with a series of allergy injections, and stopped the reactions.

Healthful hint 1: Allergy is an amazing and fascinating condition that pops up in all kinds of interesting ways.

Exercise Can Be Harmful

Dr. Albert Sheffer reported that exercise can cause hives and asthma. This made other doctors, at least it made Dr. R. Sabinsky, think about other ways exercise might be harmful. Dr. Sabinsky interviewed long distance runners after a race in New York and found almost fifty percent of them had experienced nasal symptoms during the race.

Helpful hint 1: Although regular exercise is healthy, in certain individuals exercise can produce allergic-type reactions and make you sick.

Helpful hint 2: Exercise isn't always the best thing for you.

Occupational Allergies

Hundreds of thousands of people are exposed to a bewildering array of chemicals in the workplace. Every year companies create more chemicals. Although chemicals are important for commerce and to make our lives easier, they can also cause allergy. Thousands of people are affected. Some even need to leave their jobs. Others need to take special precautions. This affects workers in all sorts of industries from pharmaceutical to agricultural to manufacturing to veterinary, and so on.

The symptoms of occupational allergy are rashes, itching, sneezing, wheezing, coughing, headaches, and fatigue. Sometimes the symptoms occur only at work. Sometimes they begin after work when the sensitized person is in the supposed safety of their home. This latter is due to *delayed-type* occupational allergy reactions.

Occupational allergy is a fascinating subject. Each industry has its own quirks. To describe all these problems in a small book would be impossible. Nevertheless you might be interested in a short list of chemicals that have been implicated in occupational allergy.

platinum salts	freon
nickel salts	sunflower pollen
trimellitic anhydride	toluene diisocyanate
mealworm	hexamethonium isocyanate
himic anhydride	poultry farm material
phthalic anhydride	moth scale
ethylene oxide	peach skin
bee pollen	

When health and safety engineers warn you about occupational exposure and its dangers, keep in mind that a toxic reaction is different from an allergic reaction. Toxic illness is due to a *high level* of a chemical that is unsafe to anyone whether he is allergic or not. For example, a high level of chlorine or acid in a swimming pool will burn, irritate, and can even cause blindness. The *normal* level of chlorine and acid is safe and actually protects you against illnesses caused by infectious organisms.

Allergy, on the other hand, occurs when a substance is present at virtually *undetectable* levels. So even if there isn't a safety or health hazard, you can still experience an allergic reaction because it is your own excess level of IgE antibody that is responsible from making you ill.

Helpful hint 1: There are a multitude of chemicals you may be exposed to at home or on the job. When present at a *high* level, these chemicals can cause *toxic* reactions in *anyone*. When present at virtually *undetectable* levels, these chemicals cause *allergic* symptoms in certain *susceptible individuals*.

Helpful hint 2: Most of the time (this is important to keep in mind) hazardous chemicals are kept to a non-hazardous level and do not cause problems.

Helpful hint 3: An allergic person's excess IgE antibody can turn a non-hazardous chemical into one that makes him ill.

Helpful hint 4: If you have symptoms at work, consult your doctor. He or she can help you decide whether or not your symptoms are work-related.

Gustatory Rhinitis

Have you ever wondered why your nose runs when you eat spicy foods?.

Dr. Michael Kaliner was curious whether this was related to allergy. Upon studying the process, Dr. Kaliner found that spicy foods contain capsaicin. Capsaicin is responsible for producing the runny nose.

Interestingly, Dr. Kaliner uses capsaicin to study nasal physiology. He needed a reliable method to stimulate mucus so he could analyze how the nose functions. If you volunteer to be a subject in his laboratory, you can eat all the spicy food you want and get paid for doing it.

Helpful hint 1: Not all runny noses are due to allergy.

Non-allergic Eosinophilic Rhinitis

Eosinophils are cells in the body which are known to be the hallmark of allergy. So when Dr. Michael Mullarkey found a group of patients who had eosinophils in their nasal mucous but had negative allergy tests, no history of allergy, and no response to anti-allergy medication, this was big news in allergy circles. This may not seem important to you, but it is to allergists.

Since many of the subjects were being treated for allergy, Dr. Mullarkey concluded that many people who are diagnosed with nasal allergy (rhinitis) may not really be allergic. As you know, allergy tends to get blamed for many events, even when it is not at fault. For example, children often say they are allergic to spinach just so they don't have to eat it.

Other reasons for *non-allergic* nasal symptoms are the common cold, overuse of nasal sprays, irritants in the air, changes in climate, certain nasal polyps, various drugs, pregnancy, and hypothyroidism.

Dr. Mullarkey's report is important because it reminds all of us, doctors and patients alike, that a *correct* diagnosis is the best hope for effective treatment.

Helpful hint 1: Not all sneezes are due to allergy.

Eye Drops Make You Worse

There are many brands of eye drops. They contain decongestants, artificial tears, antihistamines, steroids, and combinations of the above.

Dr. Sheldon Spector studied people who use the kind that contain decongestants such as Visine, Albalon-A, and Naphcon-A, to name a few. The decongestant drops contain the same type of chemical that is used in nasal decongestants.

What caught Dr. Spector's attention was that some of his patients got worse from the drops. This reminded him that people who use nasal sprays sometimes get worse from the spray.

Upon investigation, he found the adverse reaction that happens in the nose from overuse of nasal decongestant sprays was happening in the eyes. When patients first applied the drops, their eyes became whiter. However, after several applications, *certain* people developed a rebound reaction. Within a short period of time, they were using the drops several times an hour.

If you use eye drops and find you need them more and more frequently, consult your doctor.

This condition is called conjunctivitis medicamentosa. Fortunately it is uncommon. So don't be overly fearful of eye drops. Just be careful.

Helpful hint 1: Doctors have discovered a new treatment for certain cases of red, swollen, irrritated eyes. Stop using eye drops. They may be worse for you than your disease.

Copy-Paper Disease

One kind of copy paper disease is a psychological reaction to the mounds of paper that keep piling up on our desks in what the experts tell us is supposed to be a "paperless society" thanks to the wonderful world of computers. I can't help you with this problem, except to say that it seems to be getting worse and not better. Or else I'm just more sensitive to it.

On the other hand there is another copy paper disease that I can help you with. This is a reaction to copy paper itself. Since I've seen all kinds of cases in my career, I'm not usually shocked when something like this turns up. But I couldn't believe what Dr. Peter Walter reported. Copy paper has up to twenty-two chemicals in it, and Dr. Walter had to test for all twenty-two to find the one that caused the problem in one of his patients. I didn't know there was even *one* chemical in copy paper. I thought it was plain, white paper.

In this case the culprit was 2-7-Dihydroxy-naphthalene, in case you're interested.

Helpful hint 1: No matter how plain an object appears, it may be complex and contain substances you are allergic to.

Treatment For Allergy To X-Ray Contrast Material

When radiologists perform x-ray studies, they often use a substance called radiocontrast material, a chemical that illuminates your interior body organs on x-ray film. Some individuals react to the dye that is used and experience an attack of asthma, hives, or even collapse.

Dr. Roy Patterson's group in Chicago devised a method of circumventing this kind of allergic reaction. Before performing x-ray procedures with radiocontrast, Dr. Patterson gave patients several medications that are known to prevent allergic reactions. The technique has been known for many years, but Dr. Patterson did us a service by showing that the procedure is still effective.

Another way to prevent allergic reactions to radiocontrast is to use low-ion material. Many x-ray reactions are due to direct release of mast cell chemicals and not because of an allergic interaction with IgE antibody. The low-ion material can prevent this *direct-release* type of reaction.

Helpful hint 1: If you react to x-ray dye, you can still have X-rays as long as you are pretreated with certain anti-allergy medication.

Helpful hint 2: Not all hives are due to allergy. Some are due to a direct-release syndrome

Tinea And Allergy

Tinea sounds like one of those names modern, young couples give their children. It has a certain poetic ring to it.

However, Tinea is the name of a fungus that infects the skin and causes itching, peeling, and scaling. The street names are athletes foot, the itch, and so forth. It is an ugly looking disease, but it is not dangerous.

Dr. Thomas Platts-Mills from Virginia has found that Tinea can cause asthma. He treated several patients with anti-fungal drugs and even immunized several patients with fungal material. His treatment provided dramatic relief in several cases.

Helpful hint 1: In the early days of allergy, doctors immunized for infections. This became discredited, but perhaps there are certain patients where we should consider allergy to infection and treat accordingly. More studies like Dr. Platts-Mills' study will tell us what to do.

Teflon Allergy

Dr. William Shearer at Baylor Medical College treated a woman who had itching, swelling, and hives. These are classic symptoms of an allergic reaction. To find out the cause Dr. Shearer tested several substances and discovered that the Teflon coating of plastic tubes that the woman had needed for a medical treatment had caused the reaction.

You may take comfort from the fact that you aren't getting intravenous treatment with Teflon tubes, but you are probably exposed to Teflon in cooking utensils. And if Dr. Shearer's patient can develop allergy to Teflon anyone can.

Helpful hint 1: Teflon allergy is extermely rare, and you shouldn't stop eating foods cooked in Teflon-coated pans because of this one case. But this is something to think about if you seem to be reacting to foods that have no common ingredient but have been cooked in Teflon pans.

20

The Future of Allergy

Many exciting studies hold hope for alleviating allergies. Doctors are using sophisticated research and advanced equipment. Each year another piece of the puzzle falls into place.

No one can predict which, if any, of the current approaches will be the ultimate answer. But this chapter describes work that is currently in progress.

The first study describes a new substance that has been found to play a role in causing allergic reactions in humans. The hope, of course, is that an antidote could be developed against it.

The second and third studies describe techniques that might stop your body from making excessive IgE antibody.

The fourth study is a science fiction proposal to cure allergy.

Histamine Releasing Factor Has Been
Found To Be Responsible For Allergies

One of the most intensely studied subjects in allergy is how chemical mediators provoke the actual symptoms you experience.

For years doctors have known that histamine is one of the most important chemical mediators that contribute to allergic reactions. The antidote, antihistamine, ameliorates the symptoms by acting *after* histamine is already released into your tissues from cells called Mast cells. Wouldn't it be more effective if doctors could prevent histamine from being released in the first place?

Now, researchers have a better chance to accomplish this. They have discovered a substance called Histamine Releasing Factor. As the name implies, Histamine Releasing Factor is responsible for releasing histamine into your tissues. If pharmacolgists can find a drug to block the effect of Histamine Releasing Factor, this could lead to a major advance in allergy treatment.

Unfortunately it can take a long time for pharmaceutical manufacturers to develop effective drugs. Even when they do, the drug must be tested for dangerous side effects. But it is good to know that scientists have not given up the search for basic answers to allergy problems.

Exciting And Revolutionary Treatment For Allergies

At a patient's first office visit, I explain the three methods of treating allergy: avoidance, medication, and allergy injections. I also mention the last hope (and fourth choice) cortisone. Now Dr. Kimige Ishizaka, who was the first scientist to isolate IgE antibody in quantity and show that IgE was the root cause of allergy, has discovered a chemical in rats which prevents the rats from making IgE antibody. He calls it GIF which stands for glycosylation inhibiting factor.

GIF is one of a family of chemicals called Interferon. It activates certain immune cells which can then suppress the production of IgE antibody.

It is years and years too early to become optimistic about GIF. Many experiments have to be performed to confirm these initial findings. Also, we must learn whether Dr. Ishizaka's discoveries apply to humans as well as rats. And lastly, doctors must determine whether GIF is safe to use in humans. Nevertheless, someone has finally opened a crack in the door to getting directly at the manufacture of too much IgE, which is the fundamental malfunction that leads to allergy.

Helpful hint 1: Dr. Kimige Ishizaka has found a substance that may be able to turn off the manufacture of excessive IgE antibody and thus cure allergy.

Another New Treatment For Allergy

Like Dr. Ishizaka, Dr. Alec Sehon of Canada has been able to turn off IgE production in animals. He attached various allergenic proteins to a chemical called polyethylene glycol (PEG). When he injected his creation into laboratory animals, they stopped making IgE antibody for that particular allergen.

If this is going to be useful, doctors have to figure out how to attach allergens to polyethylene glycol in a safe way so that this new chemical does not create a worse disease in humans than it was meant to prevent.

A Science-Fiction Proposal For An Allergy Cure

This is a science-fiction proposal that could cure allergy with just a few injections.

As you know by now, the condition to cause allergy is created when excess IgE antibody attaches to Mast cells, thus setting your body up to react when you are exposed to various allergens. If doctors could remove the IgE from cells, they could prevent allergic symptoms from occurring. Unfortunately, removing antibodies while they are in your body is technically difficult. However, *replacing* them with another chemical is feasible.

The best substitute for IgE would be an *inactive* IgE molecule. The inactive, or false, IgE could attach to the cells, blockade the existing sites, and, being inactive, would be incapable of causing a reaction itself. Furthermore, inactive IgE is merely a modification of natural IgE and would not be a foreign chemical that might cause all sorts of undesirable side effects.

The ideal chemical for the job is the end portion of the IgE molecule itself. This portion, which is called the "Fc fragment" of IgE, is the segment of the molecule that specifically binds to IgE sites and no other sites. Therefore, the Fc fragment fulfills all the criteria for our science fiction proposal.

• The Fc fragment is a specific component of a natural substance that is already found in the body. So it is not a foreign drug.

• The Fc fragment has a strong attraction for IgE sites (scientists call this strong attraction a "high affinity"), and it is known to stick to the IgE site for long periods of time so it would not have to be replaced every few hours or even every few days.

• Finally, and most important, the Fc fragment is inactive. Thus, it could not trigger allergic reactions on its own.

On the next page is a diagram showing you how this might work.

The IgE molecule is made up of two sections. The Fc fragment is the tail and the Fab fragment is the head. If the whole IgE molecule looked like this,

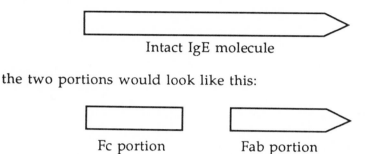

Intact IgE molecule

the two portions would look like this:

Fc portion   Fab portion

If your doctors flooded your body with blunted, inactive Fc fragments, these would bind to your Mast cells. Without a pointed Fab end, though, these molecules cannot grab onto grasses, weeds, or dust allergens. Since the allergens cannot attach to Mast cells via the IgE antibody, they would float by and be unable to trigger the release of chemical mediators like histamine. This would prevent allergic reactions.

To my knowledge, no one has done this successfully. But with the current plethora of genetic research and the amazing creation of chemicals through gene splicing, this should be possible.

A Final Word

I hope you enjoyed reading *What's New in Allergy and Asthma,* and I hope the information helps you overcome your allergy problems. However, no book can anticipate all questions. So, if you have any questions, consult your doctors and make them part of your anti-allergy team.

Appendix A

Partial List of
Drugs Used in Allergy

This is a <u>partial</u> list of the drugs used for the treatment of allergic disorders. Each drug is listed according to whether it is old, new, or super-new. If you would like a complete list of drugs, consult the *Physicians Desk Reference* which you can find in your local library. Those of you who have access to the Internet can find lists there.

Decongestants

Old   phenylephrine
phenylpropanolamine
phenyltolaxime
pseudoephedrine

Antihistamine (many contain decongestants)

Old   Atarax
                Benadryl
                Chlortrimeton
                Naldecon
                PBZ
                90 others

New   Allegra
                Astemizole
                Cetirizine
                Claritin
                Claritin-D
                Claritin-D 24 Hour
                Hismanal
                Loratidine
                Seldane
                Seldane-D
                Tavist
                Terfenadine
                Trinalin
                Zyrtec

Super-New   Azelastine
                Ebastine
                Ketotifen
                Levocobastine
                Mequitazine
                Noberastine
                Oxatomide
                Pemirolast

Sympathomimetic Bronchodilators

Old
Adrenalin
Ephedrine
Isoproterenol
Isuprel
Susphrine

New
Albuterol
Brethaire
Bricanyl
Brethine
Fenoterol
Maxair
Metaprel
Proventil
Salbutamol
Serevent
Terbutaline
Ventolin

Super-New
Berotec
Bitolterol
Formoterol
Lanetolol
Procaterol
Rotocaps
Salmeterol
Tornolate
Turbohaler

Theophylline Bronchodilators

Old   Choledyl
                   Marax*
                   Quibron
                   Slobid
                   Slophyllin
                   Tedral*
                   Theo Dur
                   UniDur
                   Uniphyl

*also contains a sympathomimetic

New   Maxivent
                   Mepiphylline
                   Monospan
                   Theo 24

Steroids

Old	Aristocort
	Decadron
	Kenalog
	Medrol
	Prednisolone
	Prednisone
New	Aerobid
	Azmacort
	Beclomethasone
	Beclovent
	Beconase
	Dexacort
	Flonase
	Flunisolide
	Nasalide
	Nasarel
	Nasacort
	Rhinocort
	Triamcinolone acetonide
	Vancenase
	Vanceril
Super-New	Budesonide
	Flovent
	Fluocortinbutyl
	Fluticosone propionate

Anti-allergic

Old	Disodium Cromoglycate
	Intal
New	Crolom
	Gastrocrom
	Lodoxamide Tromethamine
	Nasalcrom
	Opticrom
	Tilade
Super-New	Accolate
	Amlexanox
	Azelastine
	Benafentrin
	Humanized Monoclonal Antibody
	Lodoxamide Tromethamine
	Nedocromil
	Pranlukast
	Reprinast
	Rhinocrom
	Rolipram
	RO22-3747*
	Siguazodan
	Tiprinast
	Tranilast
	Zafirlukast
	Zaprinast

*also known as trans-3-[6-(methylthio)-4-oxo-4H-quinazolin-3-yl]-2-propenoic acid

Atropine-like

Old   Atrovent
                   Ipratropium Bromide
                   SCH-1000

New   Atrovent Nasal

Appendix B

Allergy Organizations, Sources of Additional Information, and Companies With Allergy Products For Sale

Allergy Organizations

American Academy of Allergy, Asthma, and Immunology
611 East Wells Street
Milwaukee, WI 53202
414-272-6071

American Allergy Association
PO Box 640
Menlo Park, CA 94026
415-322-1663

American College of Allergy, Asthma, and Immunolgy
800 E. Northwest Highway, Suite 1080
Palatine, IL 60067
708-359-2800   800-842-7777

American College of Allergists
85 West Algonquin Rd. Suite 550
Arlington Heights, IL 60005
708-427-1200

Asthma and Allergy Foundation of America
1125 15th Street N.W. Suite 502
Washington D.C. 20005
202-466-7643   800-7-ASTHMA

American Lung Association
National Headquarters
1740 Broadway,
New York, NY 10019
212-315-8700
(See the listing in your local phone book)

Food Allergy Network
4744 Holly Avenue
Fairfax, VA 22030
703-691-3179

National Allergy and Asthma Network/Mothers of Asthmatics
3554 Chain Bridge Road, Suite 2000
Fairfax, VA 22030
703-385-4403

National Jewish Center for Immunology and Respiratory Medicine
1400 Jackson Street
Denver, CO 80206
800-222-LUNG

National Institutes of Allergy and Infectious Diseases
Office of Communications
9000 Rockville Pike
Building 31, Room 7A50
Bethesda, MD 20892
301-496-5717

Companies with Products to Sell
(A listing here does not constitute endorsement)

Allergy Control Products
96 Danbury Road
Ridgefield, CT 06687
800-422-DUST

Aller/Guard, Inc.
1645 Southwest 41st St.
Topeka, KS 66609

Allergy Supply Company
P.O. Box 419
Fairfax Station VA 22039
800-323-6744

Bio-Tech Health Systems, Ltd.
4151 North Kedzie Avenue
Chicago, IL 60618

Medic Alert Foundation
2323 Colorado
Turlock, CA 95380

National Allergy Supply Company
4400 Georgia Highway 120
Duluth, GA 30136
800-522-1448

INDEX

274

Kapok, 59, 62
Ketotifen, 154
Killer bees, 223

Late onset reaction, 134
Latex allergy, 40, 244
Local Nasal Immunotherapy
 (LNIT), 130

Ma Huang, 213
MAST test, 55
Mediators, chemical, 41
Metered dose inhaler, 156,157
Methacholine test, 137
Migraine, 87
Milk allergy, 85
Minor Determinant Mixture,
230, 231
Molds, 76, 197
Monday Morning, 219
Multiple Chemical, 214

Nasal spray, 123
Night symptoms, 29

Occupational allergy, 248
Oral immunizing, 198
Osteopathy, 206
Overdose, 118

Paradoxical asthma, 138
Peak flow meter, 147
Penicillin, 227
 tests for, 230

Peptide injections, 185
Perforation, nasal, 131
Pizza, 94
Pollen, 193
Polyethylen glycol, 38
Polymerized serum, 189, 192,
Pregnancy, 233
Priming, 104
Prostaglandin, 43
Provocation test, 53
Pseudo food allergy, 87
Pulvinal, 157

Quality of life, 15

Radiocontrast material, 254
Ragweed, 196
RAST, 53, 155
Rebound, 126
Rhinitis,
Right-hand drug, 153

Salt water, 124
Seldane, 112, 115, 121
Serum, allergy, 194
Side effect, 119
Sinus disease, 102, 136
Smog, 40
Smoking, 146
Spacer, 160, 162
SRS-A, 42
STALLERZYM, 56
Steroids, 173
Sublingual test, 22
Sugar, allergy, 80

275